Radiation Therapy Planning with PET

Guest Editors

SUSHIL BERIWAL, MD
ROGER M. MACKLIS, MD
SANDIP BASU, MBBS (HONS), DRM, DNB, MNAMS

PET CLINICS

www.pet.theclinics.com

Consulting Editor
ABASS ALAVI, MD, PhD (Hon), DSc (Hon)

April 2011 • Volume 6 • Number 2

SAUNDERS an imprint of ELSEVIER, Inc.

W.B. SAUNDERS COMPANY
A Division of Elsevier Inc.

1600 John F. Kennedy Boulevard ● Suite 1800 ● Philadelphia, Pennsylvania 19103-2899

http://www.theclinics.com

PET CLINICS Volume 6, Number 2
April 2011 ISSN 1556-8598, ISBN-13: 978-1-4557-0489-7

Editor: Barton Dudlick

PET Clinics (ISSN 1556-8598) is published quarterly by Elsevier Inc., 360 Park Avenue South, New York, NY 10010-1710. Months of issue are January, April, July, and October. Periodicals postage paid at New York, NY, and additional mailing offices. Subscription prices per year are $199.00 (US individuals), $279.00 (US institutions), $102.00 (US students), $226.00 (Canadian individuals), $312.00 (Canadian institutions), $124.00 (Canadian students), $241.00 (foreign individuals), $312.00 (foreign institutions), and $124.00 (foreign students). To receive student and resident rate, orders must be accompanied by name of affiliated institution, date of term, and the signature of program/residency coordinator on institution letterhead. Orders will be billed at individual rate until proof of status is received. Foreign air speed delivery is included in all Clinics subscription prices. All prices are subject to change without notice. POSTMASTER: Send address changes to PET Clinics, Elsevier Health Sciences Division, Subscription Customer Service, 3251 Riverport Lane, Maryland Heights, MO 63043. **Customer Service: 1-800-654-2452 (U.S. and Canada); 314-447-8871 (outside U.S. and Canada). Fax: 314-447-8029. E-mail: journalscustomerservice-usa@elsevier.com (for print support); journalsonlinesupport-usa@elsevier.com (for online support).**

Reprints. For copies of 100 or more of articles in this publication, please contact the Commercial Reprints Department, Elsevier Inc., 360 Park Avenue South, New York, NY 10010-1710. Tel.: 212-633-3812; Fax: 212-462-1935; E-mail: reprints@elsevier.com.

Contributors

CONSULTING EDITOR

ABASS ALAVI, MD, PhD(Hon), DSc(Hon)
Professor of Radiology, Division of Nuclear
Medicine, University of Pennsylvania School
of Medicine, Philadelphia, Pennsylvania

GUEST EDITORS

SUSHIL BERIWAL, MD
Associate Professor, Department of Radiation
Oncology, University of Pittsburgh Cancer
Institute, Magee-Womens Hospital of UPMC,
Pittsburgh, Pennsylvania

ROGER M. MACKLIS, MD
Department of Radiation Oncology, Cleveland
Clinic Lerner College of Medicine and Taussig
Cancer Center, Cleveland, Ohio

**SANDIP BASU, MBBS (Hons), DRM, DNB,
MNAMS**
Radiation Medicine Centre (BARC), Tata
Memorial Hospital Annexe, Parel, Mumbai,
India

AUTHORS

DONALD M. CANNON, MD
Resident, Department of Human Oncology and
Radiation Oncology, University of Wisconsin
School of Medicine and Public Health,
Madison, Wisconsin

PRAJNAN DAS, MD, MS, MPH
Department of Radiation Oncology, The
University of Texas MD Anderson Cancer
Center, Houston, Texas

TIM FOX, PhD
Associate Professor, Department of Radiation
Oncology, Winship Cancer Institute, Emory
University, Atlanta, Georgia

SUSAN GUO, MD
Department of Radiation Oncology, Taussig
Cancer Center, Cleveland Clinic Lerner College
of Medicine, Cleveland, Ohio

DWIGHT E. HERON, MD, FACRO
Professor & Vice Chairman, Department of
Radiation Oncology & Otolaryngology,
University of Pittsburgh Medical Center Cancer
Pavilion, University of Pittsburgh Cancer
Institute, Pittsburgh, Pennsylvania

ANTON KHOURI, MD
Department of Radiation Oncology, University
Hospitals/Case Western Reserve University;
Case Comprehensive Cancer Center,
Cleveland, Ohio

DEEPAK KHUNTIA, MD
Associate Professor, Department of Human
Oncology and Radiation Oncology, University
of Wisconsin School of Medicine and Public
Health, Madison, Wisconsin

TIM J. KRUSER, MD
Resident, Department of Human Oncology and Radiation Oncology, University of Wisconsin School of Medicine and Public Health, Madison, Wisconsin

GREGORY J. KUBICEK, MD
Assistant Professor, Department of Radiation Oncology & Otolaryngology, University of Pittsburgh Medical Center Cancer Pavilion, University of Pittsburgh Cancer Institute, Pittsburgh, Pennsylvania

JOSH LAWSON, MD
Assistant Professor, Department of Radiation Oncology, University of California, San Diego, California

DANIEL J. MA, MD
Department of Radiation Oncology, Mallinckrodt Institute of Radiology, Siteman Cancer Center, Washington University Medical Center, St Louis, Missouri

MITCHELL MACHTAY, MD
Department of Radiation Oncology, University Hospitals/Case Western Reserve University; Case Comprehensive Cancer Center, Cleveland, Ohio

ROGER M. MACKLIS, MD
Professor of Medicine, Department of Radiation Oncology, Taussig Cancer Center, Cleveland Clinic Lerner College of Medicine, Cleveland, Ohio

TINSU PAN, PhD
Department of Imaging Physics, The University of Texas MD Anderson Cancer, Houston, Texas

EDUARD SCHREIBMANN, PhD
Assistant Professor, Department of Radiation Oncology, Winship Cancer Institute, Emory University, Atlanta, Georgia

SHETAL N. SHAH, MD
Departments of Abdominal Imaging and Nuclear Medicine; Co-director, Center for PET and Molecular Imaging, Imaging Institute, Cleveland Clinic, Cleveland, Ohio

JASON SOHN, PhD
Associate Professor, Department of Radiation Oncology, University Hospitals Case Medical Center, Case Western Reserve University School of Medicine, Cleveland, Ohio

SHYAM M. SRINIVAS, MD, PhD
Department of Nuclear Medicine; Co-director, Center for PET and Molecular Imaging, Imaging Institute, Cleveland Clinic, Cleveland, Ohio

KEVIN STEPHANS, MD
Department of Radiation Oncology, Cleveland Clinic; Case Comprehensive Cancer Center, Cleveland, Ohio

STEPHANIE A. TEREZAKIS, MD
Assistant Professor, Department of Radiation Oncology and Molecular Radiation Sciences, Johns Hopkins School of Medicine, Baltimore, Maryland

CHIAOJUNG JILLIAN TSAI, MD, PhD
Department of Radiation Oncology, The University of Texas MD Anderson Cancer Center, Houston, Texas

CHARLES WOODS, MD
Resident, Department of Radiation Oncology, University Hospitals Case Medical Center, Case Western Reserve University School of Medicine, Cleveland, Ohio

JOACHIM YAHALOM, MD
Professor, Department of Radiation Oncology, Memorial Sloan-Kettering Cancer Center, New York, New York

MIN YAO, MD, PhD
Associate Professor, Department of Radiation Oncology, University Hospitals Case Medical Center, Case Western Reserve University School of Medicine, Cleveland, Ohio

HABIB ZAIDI, PhD, PD
Division of Nuclear Medicine, Geneva University Hospital; Geneva Neuroscience Center, Geneva University, Geneva, Switzerland

Contents

> PET scans are becoming increasingly used in oncology and especially radiation oncology. While the potential and indicated uses continue to grow, so do the data and evidence to support the growing use. This article summarizes the physics behind PET-computed tomographic (CT) scans, how PET scans fit into the treatment paradigms for patients with cancer including staging, assessment of response, and identifying the prognostic features, with a special emphasis on the role of PET-CT scans in radiation therapy planning.

> PET/computed tomography (CT) has been used for both diagnosis/ staging of cancer and guiding the cancer treatment planning process. PET-guided radiotherapy (RT) planning has been increasingly used to assist in determining the tumor locations so that therapy procedures can be focused on the tumor, minimizing damage to the surrounding tissue. However, incorporating PET/CT into the treatment planning process raises challenges in areas of immobilization, image registration, and target volume segmentation. This article focuses on the technical aspects of integrating PET/CT into radiotherapy planning and presents a general overview of the clinical workflow and challenges involved in the planning.

> For tumors of the central nervous system (CNS), the ability to accurately delineate the extent of tumor has implications for diagnosis, prognosis, and treatment. PET, mainly with ^{18}F-fluorodeoxyglucose (FDG), has become commonplace in the work-up of many extracranial tumors. However, the relative high background of FDG-PET activity of normal brain tissue has limited the applicability of this modality in CNS tumors to date. More recently, novel PET tracers for imaging of CNS tumors have been developed. This article outlines recent advances in PET as a complementary imaging modality with implications for diagnosis, prognosis, surgical and radiation treatment planning, and post-therapy surveillance in malignancies of the CNS. Pharmacokinetic properties of the radiotracers and the influence of blood-brain-barrier integrity are also incorporated into the discussion.

> Radiation treatment plays an important role in the management of head and neck cancer, for which planning is critical in delineating the target volumes. ^{18}F-fluoro-deoxy-D-glucose PET is being using increasingly in oncologic imaging as a useful

tool for target delineation of tumors in treatment planning for radiotherapy as well as in the management of head and neck cancers. PET is now routinely used in the staging of head and neck cancer because of to its improved accuracy. This article provides an overview of how ^{18}F -fluoro-deoxy-D-glucose PET imaging is being used in the context of radiation treatment planning for head and neck cancers. The use of PET imaging in conjunction with treatment planning CT data can significantly change radiation treatment plans. Current techniques for image registration, target delineation, image segmentation, and the use new radiotracers and dose escalation are explored as well as current challenges and limitations of the technology.

FDG-PET is an extremely useful tool for staging and response assessment in multiple malignancies including lymphoma and hematologic malignancies. Its growing importance in radiation treatment planning has also been demonstrated in multiple studies. However, there are many potential pitfalls of PET, particularly in radiation planning, and radiation oncologists must be mindful of the complexities of PET before adapting it for routine use. Close collaboration with nuclear medicine is essential to appropriately interpret PET findings for the design of radiation treatment volumes for lymphoma patients. Long-term clinical outcomes are needed to determine the effect of PET in radiation planning.

PET has gained a major role in the evaluation and treatment of lung cancer over the past two decades. Over that time span PET and treatment techniques have both evolved substantially. While technical changes in PET and PET/computed tomography have improved accuracy and reliability, the evolution toward increasingly targeted and intensive treatment has increased the reliance upon imaging of radiation treatment. This article seeks to review the current role of PET in the evaluation and treatment of lung cancer with radiation.

Many studies have explored the use of ^{18}F-flurodeoxyglucose (FDG-PET) with CT for radiation therapy planning. The addition of PET/CT could improve tumor volume delineation, reduce geographic misses, and decrease treatment-related toxicity. For cancers of the gastrointestinal tract, the potential benefit of FDG-PET in radiation therapy management is less frequently studied. This article reviews the literature concerning PET/CT in radiation treatment planning. PET/CT appears to have an impact on tumor volume definition. More studies are needed to determine the impact of PET/CT-based radiation therapy on local control, patterns of failure, and treatment-related toxicity.

In addition to allowing much greater technical precision, the modern era allows investigation of target physiology and it is the potential incorporation of physiologic information into the treatment-planning rubric that gives modern PET-CT its allure and promise. Although oncologic PET scanning has been clinically available for more than 10 years, it is only recently that sufficient investigative and retrospective data have become available to confidently assert that future radiotherapy treatment planning will include functional imaging as an obligatory dimension of clinical characterization for most gynecologic tumors. This article explores the role of functional imaging in radiotherapy planning and management of gynecologic malignancies.

In the past decade, there have been many contributions demonstrating the advantages of combining morphologic and molecular imaging, and with commercial PET/CT scanners emerging in the same time frame, PET/CT has already had a significant impact on patient management. Ultimately, molecular imaging-guided radiotherapy holds the promise of improved definition of tumor target volumes. Yet, despite considerable progress to date, challenges remain if the potential of PET/CT-guided radiotherapy treatment planning is to be fully exploited in clinics.

PET Clinics

THE CLINICS ARE NOW AVAILABLE ONLINE!

Access your subscription at:
www.theclinics.com

GOAL STATEMENT

The goal of the *PET Clinics* is to keep practicing radiologists and radiology residents up to date with current clinical practice in positron emission tomography by providing timely articles reviewing the state of the art in patient care.

ACCREDITATION

PET Clinics is planned and implemented in accordance with the Essential Areas and Policies of the Accreditation Council for Continuing Medical Education (ACCME) through the joint sponsorship of the University of Virginia School of Medicine and Elsevier. The University of Virginia School of Medicine is accredited by the ACCME to provide continuing medical education for physicians.

The University of Virginia School of Medicine designates this educational activity for a maximum of 15 *AMA PRA Category 1 Credits*™ for each issue, 60 credits per year. Physicians should only claim credit commensurate with the extent of their participation in the activity.

The American Medical Association has determined that physicians not licensed in the US who participate in this CME activity are eligible for a maximum of 15 *AMA PRA Category 1 Credits*™ for each issue, 60 credits per year.

Category 1 credit can be earned by reading the text material, taking the CME examination online at http://www.theclinics.com/home/cme, and completing the evaluation. After taking the test, you will be required to review any and all incorrect answers. Following completion of the test and evaluation, your credit will be awarded and you may print your certificate.

FACULTY DISCLOSURE/CONFLICT OF INTEREST

The University of Virginia School of Medicine, as an ACCME accredited provider, endorses and strives to comply with the Accreditation Council for Continuing Medical Education (ACCME) Standards of Commercial Support, Commonwealth of Virginia statutes, University of Virginia policies and procedures, and associated federal and private regulations and guidelines on the need for disclosure and monitoring of proprietary and financial interests that may affect the scientific integrity and balance of content delivered in continuing medical education activities under our auspices.

The University of Virginia School of Medicine requires that all CME activities accredited through this institution be developed independently and be scientifically rigorous, balanced and objective in the presentation/discussion of its content, theories and practices.

All authors/editors participating in an accredited CME activity are expected to disclose to the readers relevant financial relationships with commercial entities occurring within the past 12 months (such as grants or research support, employee, consultant, stock holder, member of speakers bureau, etc.). The University of Virginia School of Medicine will employ appropriate mechanisms to resolve potential conflicts of interest to maintain the standards of fair and balanced education to the reader. Questions about specific strategies can be directed to the Office of Continuing Medical Education, University of Virginia School of Medicine, Charlottesville, Virginia.

The faculty and staff of the University of Virginia Office of Continuing Medical Education have no financial affiliations to disclose.

The authors/editors listed below have identified no professional or financial affiliations for themselves or their spouse/partner:

Abass Alavi, MD(Hon), PhD(Hon), DSc(Hon) (Consulting Editor); Sandip Basu, MBBS (Hons), DRM, DNB, MNAMS (Guest Editor); Sushil Beriwal, MD (Guest Editor); Donald M. Cannon, MD; Barton Dudlick (Acquisitions Editor); Susan Guo, MD; Dwight E. Heron, MD, FACRO; Anton Khouri, MD; Tim J. Kruser, MD; Gregory J. Kubicek, MD; Daniel J. Ma, MD; Mitchell Machtay, MD; Patrice Rehm, MD (Test Editor); Eduard Schreibmann, PhD; Shetal N. Shah, MD; Jason Sohn, PhD; Kevin Stephans, MD; Stephanie A. Terezakis, MD; Chiaojung Jillian Tsai, MD, PhD; Charles Woods, MD; Joachim Yahalom, MD; Min Yao, PhD; and Habib Zaidi, MD, PhD.

The authors/editors listed below identified the following professional or financial affiliations for themselves or their spouse/partner:

Prajnan Das, MD, MS, MPH is an industry funded research/investigator for Genetech.

Tim Fox, PhD is on the Advisory Board, receives royalties, and owns stock for Velocity Medical Solutions; is an industry funded research/investigator for Varian Medical Systems; and is on the Advisory Board for General Electric.

Deepak Khuntia, MD is on the Speakers' Bureau for Tomotherapy, Inc, is a consultant for Procertus, Inc, and is on the Advisory Committee/Board for Radion Global.

Josh Lawson, MD receives honoraria from Varian Medical Systems.

Roger M. Macklis, MD (Guest Editor) is on the Speakers' Bureau for Citigroup new technology forum.

Tinsu Pan, PhD is an industry funded research/investigator for Varian Medical Systems.

Shyam M. Srinivas, MD, PhD is an industry funded research/investigator and is on the Advisory Committee/Board for Siemens Molecular Imaging.

Disclosure of Discussion of Non-FDA Approved Uses for Pharmaceutical Products and/or Medical Devices.

The University of Virginia School of Medicine, as an ACCME provider, requires that all faculty presenters identify and disclose any off-label uses for pharmaceutical and medical device products. The University of Virginia School of Medicine recommends that each physician fully review all the available data on new products or procedures prior to clinical use.

TO ENROLL

To enroll in the PET Clinics Continuing Medical Education program, call customer service at 1-800-654-2452 or visit us online at www.theclinics.com/home/cme. The CME program is available to subscribers for an additional fee of $196.00.

GOAL STATEMENT

The goal of this PET Clinics is to keep practicing radiologists and radiology residents up to date with current clinical practice in positron emission tomography by providing timely articles reviewing the state of the art in their field.

ACCREDITATION

PET Clinics is planned and implemented in accordance with the essential areas and policies of the Accreditation Council for Continuing Medical Education (ACCME) through the joint sponsorship of the University of Virginia School of Medicine and Elsevier. The University of Virginia School of Medicine is accredited by the ACCME to provide continuing medical education for physicians.

The University of Virginia School of Medicine designates this educational activity for a maximum of 15 AMA PRA Category 1 Credits™ for each issue, 60 credits per year. Physicians should only claim credit commensurate with the extent of their participation in the activity.

The American Medical Association has determined that physicians not licensed in the US who participate in this CME activity are eligible for a maximum of 15 AMA PRA Category 1 Credits™ for each issue, 60 credits per year.

Credit can be earned by reading the text material, taking the CME examination online at http://www.theclinics.com/home/cme, and completing the evaluation. After taking the test, you will be required to review any and all incorrect answers. Following completion of the test and evaluation, your credit will be awarded and you may print your certificate.

FACULTY DISCLOSURE/CONFLICT OF INTEREST

The University of Virginia School of Medicine, as an ACCME accredited provider, endorses and strives to comply with the Accreditation Council for Continuing Medical Education (ACCME) Standards of Commercial Support, Commonwealth of Virginia statutes, University of Virginia policies and procedures, and associated federal and private regulations and guidelines on the need for disclosure and monitoring of proprietary and financial interests that may affect the scientific integrity and balance of content delivered in continuing medical education activities under our sponsorship.

The University of Virginia School of Medicine requires that all CME activities accredited through this institution be developed independently and be scientifically rigorous, balanced and objective in the presentation/discussion of its content, theories and practices.

All authors/editors participating in an accredited CME activity are expected to disclose to the audience any relevant financial relationships with commercial interests whose products or devices may be mentioned in the CME activity, or with the commercial supporter of the CME activity. The intent of this disclosure is not to prevent a speaker with a financial, commercial, or professional interest from participating in the activity, but rather to provide listeners with information on which they can make their own judgments. It remains for the audience to determine whether the speaker's interests or relationships may influence the presentation with regard to exposition or conclusion.

The faculty and staff of the University of Virginia Office of Continuing Medical Education have no financial affiliations to disclose.

The authors/editors listed below have identified no professional or financial affiliations for themselves or their spouse/partner:

The authors/editors listed below identified the following professional or financial affiliations for themselves or their spouse/partner:

Disclosure of Discussion of Non-FDA Approved Uses for Pharmaceutical Products and/or Medical Devices

The University of Virginia School of Medicine, as an ACCME provider, requires that all faculty presenters identify and disclose any off-label uses for pharmaceutical and medical device products. The University of Virginia School of Medicine recommends that each physician fully review all the available data on new products or procedures prior to instituting use.

TO ENROLL

To enroll in the PET Clinics Continuing Medical Education program, call customer service at 1-800-654-2452 or visit us online at www.theclinics.com/home/cme. The CME program is available to subscribers for an additional fee of $196.00.

Preface
Radiation Therapy Planning with PET

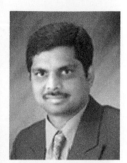

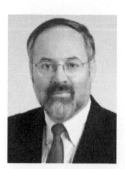

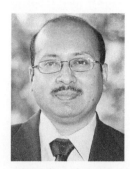

Sushil Beriwal, MD   Roger M. Macklis, MD   Sandip Basu, MBBS (Hons), DRM, DNB, MNAMS

Guest Editors

Radiation therapy planning has traditionally relied on anatomical imaging with CT scan. In recent times, there has been tremendous enthusiasm in the use of PET-guided radiation therapy planning. The advent of dual-modality integrated PET/CT systems offers a unique opportunity of improving target localization and facilitating treatment planning for radiation therapy. One distinct advantage of PET/CT in radiotherapy planning is its potential for improving tumor delineation, reducing intra-observer and interobserver variability, and making treatment volumes more standard across individuals and institutions. But incorporation of PET into three-dimensional radiation therapy planning is technically challenging and requires careful attention to detail. The use of PET/CT for target volume selection should be considered within the framework of its sensitivity and specificity for various tumor types and also mandates specific tuning of parameters, such as image acquisition, processing, and segmentation.

In this framework, in this special issue of *PET Clinics*, we are covering the advantages, indications, and pitfalls of PET/CT planning by the leaders in the field. It starts with a clinical and technical overview of the PET/CT for RT planning and issues associated with it. This is followed by systematic review on the use of PET for the main tumor sites, including lung cancer, brain tumors, head and neck cancer, lung cancer, gynecological cancer, gastrointestinal cancer, and lymphoma. Last, the ongoing

advancement in the field of nuclear imaging with different isotopes and their implication for RT planning in future are reviewed.

The goals of this issue are to provide comprehensive in-depth review of this subject and to serve as a useful guide for clinicians in deciding and optimizing the use of PET/CT in radiation planning for various malignancies.

Sushil Beriwal, MD
Department of Radiation Oncology
University of Pittsburgh Cancer Institute
Magee-Womens Hospital of UPMC
300 Halket Street
Pittsburgh, PA 15213, USA

Roger M. Macklis, MD
Department of Radiation Oncology
Cleveland Clinic Lerner College of Medicine
and Taussig Cancer Center
9500 Euclid Avenue
Cleveland, OH 44195, USA

Sandip Basu, MBBS (Hons), DRM, DNB, MNAMS
Radiation Medicine Centre (BARC)
Tata Memorial Hospital Annexe
Parel, Mumbai 400012,
India

E-mail addresses:
beriwals@upmc.edu (S. Beriwal)
macklir@ccf.org (R.M. Macklis)
drsanb@yahoo.com (S. Basu)

PET Clin 6 (2011) xi
doi:10.1016/j.cpet.2011.03.002

Clinical Applications of PET-Computed Tomography in Planning Radiotherapy: General Principles and an Overview

Gregory J. Kubicek, MD, Dwight E. Heron, MD*

KEYWORDS

• PET-CT • Treatment planning • Simulation • Outcomes

PET scans are becoming increasingly used in oncology and especially radiation oncology. While the potential and indicated uses continue to grow, so do the data and evidence to support the growing use. This article summarizes the physics behind PET-computed tomographic (CT) scans, how PET scans fit into the treatment paradigms for patients with cancer including staging, assessment of response, and identifying the prognostic features, with a special emphasis on the role of PET-CT scans in radiation therapy planning. Equally important is a discussion of several issues of PET-CT in radiotherapy planning that are yet to be resolved such as the best method of converting PET-CT data into radiation therapy treatment volumes and the effect of respiratory motion.

PHYSICS OF PET

PET scans function by the emission and collection of positrons. Certain unstable radioisotopes (such as fluorine 18 [^{18}F]) undergo a type of radioactive decay known as positron emission (also referred to as beta decay). In this type of decay, the radioisotope spontaneously emits a positron. Positrons are the highly unstable antiparticles of electrons, and after traveling only a few millimeters, a positron encounters an electron with which it combines. This encounter destroys both the electron and the positron and in their place produces a pair of annihilation (511 keV gamma) photons, which always leave the site of reaction traveling in exactly opposite directions (180° from each other). The photons are collected by the PET scan device, which can use the timing and location of the collected annihilation photons to calculate where the positron emission occurred. After a large number of such events, it becomes possible to determine which areas had more radioisotope accumulation (which in turn leads to more positron emission events).

Radioisotopes that decay by positron emission can be combined with clinically useful molecules for imaging; the combination of the molecule with the radioisotope is referred to as a radiopharmaceutical. The amounts of radiolabeled material administered are extremely small (10^{-6}–10^{-9} g) and have essentially no meaningful radiation dose; the dose of radiation given off by the radiopharmaceuticals does not have any therapeutic effect.

The foundation of PET clinical utility is based on the disproportionate accumulation of a PET scan radiopharmaceutical between different types of

Department of Radiation Oncology & Otolaryngology, University of Pittsburgh Cancer Institute, Pittsburgh, PA, USA
* Corresponding author. UPMC Cancer Pavilion, 5150 Centre Avenue, Suite 545, Pittsburgh, PA 15232.
E-mail address: herond2@upmc.edu

PET Clin 6 (2011) 105–115
doi:10.1016/j.cpet.2011.02.003

tissues. In terms of oncology, it has been known since the 1920s that cancer cells exhibit an increased rate of glycolysis[1] relative to normal cells. This increase in glycolysis corresponds to the cancer cells requiring more glucose. Fluoro-2-deoxy-D-glucose is molecularly similar to normal glucose but with some important differences. Fluoro-2-deoxy-D-glucose is able to be transported intracellularly by membrane-bound glucose transport mechanism and phosphorylated by hexokinase to a larger molecule, fluoro-glucose-6-phosphate (PO_4) in direct proportion to the glycolytic rate of the cell (which views fluoro-2-deoxy-D-glucose as regular glucose). Unlike the normal metabolite of glucose (glucose-6-PO_4), fluoro-glucose-6-PO_4 cannot enter the glycolytic pathway and steadily accumulates in the intracellular compartment of the cell. Fluoro-2-deoxy-D-glucose can easily be made to incorporate an unstable isotope of fluorine ^{18}F. ^{18}F is an unsteady isotope that decays via positron emission. The combination of 2-deoxy-D-glucose with ^{18}F (2-deoxy-D-glucose labeled with ^{18}F or FDG) is what allows PET scans to detect the differential degree of glycolysis present in a variety of tissues.

There is an infinite number of theoretical PET scan radioisotopes. All that is required is for a substance that can be radiolabeled with an isotope that decays by positron emission (such as ^{18}F, 15C). This substance must have disproportionate accumulation in tissues that are to be differentiated via the PET scan. Although novel PET markers are continuing to be evaluated and tested clinically, at present the most commonly used (and sometimes synonymous) radioisotope in PET scanning is ^{18}F FDG. In theory, any molecule that can be modified or tagged with a radioactive probe could serve as a PET scan radiopharmaceutical.

Standard uptake value (SUV) is another important concept in PET scan physics. SUV is the amount of detected radiotracer uptake in a region relative to the background radiotracer uptake. SUV can be reported in several ways, it is typically reported as a maximum value (ie, SUV of 19), which is defined by the pixel within a region of interest that exhibits the greatest SUV. The utility of SUV is debated because some think that there is too much variability between PET scan SUV values and that PET scans should simply be interpreted as being positive or negative.[2] Others find an objective value to be useful and find the absolute level of SUV to be prognostic.

PET TECHNOLOGY

PET scans are becoming increasingly used in oncology because they provide unique information not supplied by other anatomic-based imaging methods, such as CT or MR imaging scans. PET provides information on the functional nature of the tissue being examined. PET technology has been available for more than 30 years but has only become a major clinical factor in the last 10 to 15 years. The growing availability of PET is due to several causes including dramatic improvements in technology, the routine availability of medical cyclotrons (to produce the necessary short-lived positron emitters), and favorable reimbursement decisions in the late 1990s. Although PET scans are predominantly used in oncology, other fields of medicine including cardiology and neurology are also beginning to use PET scan technology.

A large factor in the increase in PET scan utility is the integration of PET and CT scans. Dual-modality techniques offer an advantage over separately obtained CT and PET scans in correlating functional and anatomic images without requiring the patient to have 2 separate scans. This technique combined the best of both imaging technologies; it produces anatomic and functional images with the patient in the same position and during a single procedure. Dual-modality imaging offers several potential advantages over conventional imaging techniques. First, the PET and x-ray CT images are complimentary to one another. PET images can identify areas of disease that are not apparent on the CT images alone. CT scans provide an anatomic correlation that can differentiate normal radiotracer uptake from that indicating disease and also more precisely localize disease sites within the body. Second, the low-noise x-ray CT data can be used to generate attenuation information, which improves the PET emission data in terms of photon attenuation,[3] scattered radiation,[4] and other physical degrading factors such as partial volume effect.[3] In these ways, the CT images can be used to improve both the visual quality and the quantitative accuracy of the PET scan data.[5–10]

The next technological breakthrough in terms of PET scan is in incorporating the CT scan used in radiation treatment planning (RTP) with the PET scan. Before beginning a course of radiotherapy, patients have a CT simulation for RTP. Although very similar to a diagnostic CT scan, the CT simulation for RTP is different in that the patient must be positioned the same way he or she will be positioned for the daily radiation treatments. Although a PET and radiation therapy planning CT scans could be performed separately and combined, there are certain advantages to having a PET-CT simulation. PET-CT simulators are a single platform that has both PET and CT capabilities, allowing the patient to have a PET scan in the radiation therapy planning position. This allows for seamless incorporation of PET scan information into radiation therapy planning and is at the same time convenient for the patient. Although this technology is not available everywhere, it is becoming more widespread.

CLINICAL APPLICATION OF PET-CT

The first major use of PET scans was in diagnostic radiology. With this novel technology, it became possible to determine the metabolic activity of tissues and thus differentiate normal tissue from a malignant one, which continues to be a major role of PET scans. Concurrent with the improvement in PET scan technology, there has been a rapid improvement in therapeutic radiologic technology. Intensity-modulated radiation therapy (IMRT) and image-guided radiation therapy (IGRT) have allowed for higher doses of radiation to be safely given to smaller areas.[1,11–14] In non-IMRT radiation techniques (eg, opposed laterals in the treatment of head and neck cancer [HNC]), there was no way to spare tissues that were next to the target volume. IMRT overcomes this limitation by using a large number of radiation beams (beamlets) of different intensities and coming from different directions (**Fig. 1**). With IMRT, it becomes increasingly important to have a more accurate definition of the target volume, and thus a growing relationship between therapeutic radiation and diagnostic imaging. PET scans have been an important step in this direction.

Although PET scans are used in a variety of ways and for a variety of diseases, PET scan utility can be thought of in terms of staging and prognosis, predictive value, and RTP.

PET Scans for Staging and Prognosis

Staging and prognosis is the most commonly thought of use for PET scans. The ability to more accurately determine the extent of disease through the use of metabolic imaging has allowed delivery of better therapy to patients. Patients who would have been considered to have local disease but are found on PET scan to have distant disease are spared toxic therapy that would be of little benefit. Similarly, patients with questionable sites of distant disease who are found on PET scan to have only local disease can be referred for aggressive and curative therapy.

PET scans have been shown to upstage patients (ie, find distant metastatic disease) in a variety of oncology settings. For example, in anal cancer, several recent series[15–17] have shown that PET scans will identify metastatic lymph nodes in 17% to 24% of patients who were radiographically node negative on CT scan. Another study[17] found that PET scans changed anal cancer staging in 23% of patients. In lung cancer, PET has proved invaluable in the initial assessment of a solitary pulmonary nodule, with the sensitivity and specificity of FDG-PET approaching 90%.[18,19]

It should be noted that PET scan does have some limitations in terms of staging and prognosis. Although PET scans are good at detecting distant disease not appreciated with other imaging modalities, PET is also prone to false-positive

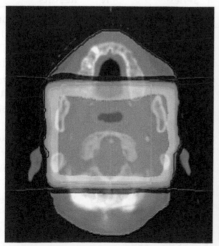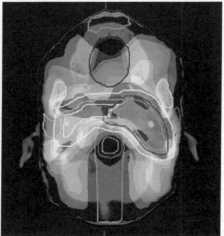

Fig. 1. Example of radiotherapy dose distribution using conventional and IMRT treatment plans. Conventional and IMRT dose plans for the same patient show the decreased area of high doses (*red and orange*) with the IMRT plan but an increase in the volume of tissue receiving lower doses (*blue and green*).

results. False-positive findings occur most commonly with infectious or inflammatory tissue that causes an increase in metabolism and thus an uptake of ^{18}F FDG.[20] [18]F FDG has been reported to accumulate in various inflammatory processes.[21–23] One often-confusing scenario is increased PET uptake seen in tissue after radiation therapy. Inflammatory changes after radiation therapy can look very similar (if not absolutely identical) to active cancer. Also, ^{18}F FDG uptake can vary widely in normal tissue, and regions of discrete uptake in areas such as the ureters, bowel, lymphatic tissue, thymus, brown fat, and muscle can be misinterpreted as abnormal. A mild to moderate increase in ^{18}F FDG uptake can also be seen in a variety of benign processes, many of which represent inflammatory or hyperplastic conditions (eg, villous adenomas, thyroid adenomas, Graves disease, adrenal adenoma, Paget disease, and fibrous dysplasia). It is important that distant metastatic disease seen on PET scan be proven by biopsy if a false-positive PET scan result would change patient management.

PET Scans as Surrogates for Clinical Outcome

Although stage remains a significant prognostic factor, PET scan information may have further prognostic ability above and beyond staging. Aggressive cancers are hypothesized to be metabolically active, which in turn leads to a higher SUV on the PET scan. Several series have shown that PET scans may be prognostic in lung and head and neck malignancies (**Tables 1** and **2**). Although knowing the prognosis is useful, actually altering and improving the prognosis is of more value. Predictive value is the ability of a test to predict how a patient will respond to treatment. For example, in non–small cell lung carcinoma (NSCLC), an SUV of 20 in a lung lesion carries a worse prognosis than an SUV of less than 20. A predictive feature would be that this lesion with a higher SUV is more likely to respond to a triple chemotherapy regimen than a lung lesion with an SUV of less than 20. Predictive factors are in general much more difficult to derive than prognostic factors because they take clinical interventions and longer follow-up to demonstrate.

Currently, there are few predictive uses for PET scans. Several studies[24] have shown that a lymph node SUV greater than 10 is prognostic for an increased risk of distant metastatic disease in HNC. Induction chemotherapy has been hypothesized to decrease the risk of distant metastatic disease, and thus it is possible that lymph node SUV can be viewed as a prognostic factor in terms of being able to stratify and predict patients who will

have a good response to induction chemotherapy for HNC. Furthermore, there is early evidence suggesting that change in SUV in lung cancer can accurately predict survival in patients with lung cancer.[25] More work needs to be done to validate existing predictive PET factors and establish more.

Table 1
Prognostic ability of PET in HNC

Series	N	Results
Roh et al,[63] 2007	79	SUV >8 → worse DFS (P = .007)
Kubicek et al,[64] 2007	212	SUV >8 → worse OS (P = .014)
Schwartz et al,[65] 2004	54	SUV >9.0 → worse DFS (P = .03)
Allal et al,[66] 2004	120	SUV >4.75 → worse DFS (P = .005)
Kitagawa et al,[67] 2003	20	SUV >7.0 → less likely CR
Halfpenny et al,[68] 2002	58	SUV >10.0 → worse survival (P = .003)
Brun et al,[69] 2002	47	SUV >9.0 → worse LRC (P = .002)
Greven et al,[70] 2001	45	SUV not predictive
Minn et al,[71] 1997	37	SUV >9.0 → worse DFS

Abbreviations: CR, complete response; DFS, disease-free survival; LRC, locoregional control; OS, overall survival.

Table 2
Prognostic ability of PET in non–small cell lung carcinoma

Series	N	Results
Van Baardwijk et al,[72] 2007	102	SUV >8 → worse OS (only stage I and II)
Vesselle et al,[73] 2007	208	SUV not predictive
Cerfolio et al,[74] 2005	315	SUV predicts for worse OS in IB–IIIA
Downey et al,[75] 2004	100	SUV >9 → worse OS
Jeong et al,[76] 2002	73	SUV >7.0 → worse survival
Higashi et al,[77] 2002	57	SUV >5.0 → worse DFS
Vansteenkiste et al,[78] 1999	125	SUV >7.0 → worse survival
Okereke et al,[79] 2009	512	SUV >12.5 → worse OS

Abbreviations: DFS, disease-free survival; OS, overall survival.

PET Scans and RTP

The third major use of PET scans is in assisting in RTP. More contemporary treatment technologies, such as IMRT and stereotactic body radiosurgery, use much more conformal radiation delivery techniques than previous radiotherapy technologies. These new technologies allow for higher radiation doses to the tumor and less radiation to the normal structures but have less tolerance of error; if the target areas are not defined precisely, the radiation all together misses the intended target. Furthermore, the ability to distinguish tumor from normal tissue is important in further being able to decrease normal tissue toxicity. For these reasons, PET scans are becoming increasingly important in RTP.

PET scans are being used in several treatment sites; the following sections detail the use of PET scan technology in individual cancer sites.

PET scans and RTP: lung cancer

Treatment of the primary lung cancer is often complicated by associated atelectasis. In this setting, it is often difficult to distinguish the tumor from surrounding reactive but normal tissues. Traditionally, the entire abnormality was uniformly irradiated because there was no way of differentiating collapsed lung from tumor. The result of this approach was further compromise of pulmonary function along with the associated increased risk of radiation-induced pneumonitis. **Fig. 2** shows a clinical example of how PET scan is able to exclude atelectatic lung from the radiation field.

In addition to allowing the radiation plan to exclude areas of atelectasis, PET scans are also useful in being able to include or exclude lymph node regions. One of the major deterrents to using higher radiation doses in lung cancer (which are thought to provide a higher likelihood of cancer cure) is the volume of normal lung tissue in the radiation field. Inclusion of noncancerous mediastinum regions are in the radiation field drastically increases the lung dose and decreases the dose to the tumor. In evaluating the mediastinum, the negative predicative values for PET is 90%.[26–29] Thus, if the mediastinal lymph node regions are not PET avid, they can safely be omitted form the radiation field. Several series have looked at the effect on radiation treatment fields when PET scan information is incorporated, and some reports have shown significant alterations in the treatment design in up to 50% of patients.[30]

PET scans and RTP: HNC

PET scans have played an important role in head and neck radiotherapy planning.[3,4,31–34] Geets and colleagues[35] reported that the use of pretreatment FDG-PET in combination with pretreatment CT or MR imaging improves target definition in oropharyngeal cancer and results in more normal tissue sparing. The same group also examined the role of PET contouring in larynx cancer by comparing standard imaging techniques and PET findings with the pathologic specimens.[36] They reported significantly smaller target volumes when the targets were drawn on FDG-PET as opposed to CT scan. PET-based tumor volumes also showed better correlation with pathologic findings compared with CT, both for the primary tumor and the locoregional lymph nodes.[36] Long-term clinical data are emerging; favorable 3-year overall state and disease-free survival rates have been reported in patients with HNC treated with IMRT, all of who had PET-based contouring.[37]

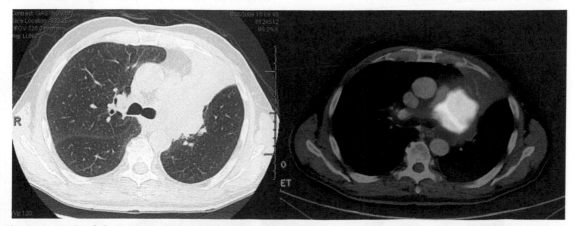

Fig. 2. Example of the use a PET-CT scan to differentiate atelectasis from tumor. Whereas atelectasis and tumor look identical on the CT scan (*left*), the PET-CT (*right*) scan shows the tumor to be metabolically active, although the atelectasis does not have any increase in metabolic activity. In this way, the size of the radiation field can be decreased.

PET scans and RTP: esophageal and gastrointestinal cancers

Combined chemoradiotherapy, with or without surgery, is commonly used to treat esophageal carcinoma. PET can improve the accuracy of radiation therapy planning mostly through better target definition.[38] CT scans, especially with barium contrast, are good at determining the radial extent of the tumor. However, CT scans are less useful in lymph node metastases and also less useful in determining the longitudinal extent of the tumor. PET, however, is able to overcome these deficiencies. PET scan is more accurate than CT for nodal assessment,[39] except for nodes that lie adjacent to the esophagus (which are obscured by the uptake of the esophageal primary itself). PET scan also shows the longitudinal extent of the tumor better than CT. Furthermore, large and bulky tumors can often make visual inspection of the primary tumor impossible. In these situations, PET may be the only way to visualize the lower border of the tumor. Several studies have shown that PET technology can improve radiation target accuracy and prevent geographic misses.[40,41] PET scans have also been used to assist in designing the radiation fields in anal cancer. Multiple series in anal cancer[17,42,43] have found that PET scan alters radiation treatment fields in up to 25% of patients treated for gastrointestinal malignancies.

PET scans and RTP: gynecologic cancers

PET scans can assist in the treatment of cervical cancers by helping to detect positive pelvic and para-aortic lymph nodes.[44–47] Detection of lymph nodes in combination with improvement in definition of the primary target affects IMRT planning.[48,49] Also, PET has been used to assist in target definition for brachytherapy.[50]

POTENTIAL PITFALLS AND UNSETTLED ISSUES IN PET SCAN RADIATION PLANNING

There are multiple issues that need to be further defined in PET scan–assisted treatment planning. Some of these issues include how to incorporate separately obtained PET scan data, what is the optimal way to define tumors with PET scans, and how to account for respiratory motion.

Issue 1: Separately Acquired Scans

The first of these issues is how to best incorporate PET information into the radiation therapy planning scan. Ideally, a PET/CT dedicated to RTP should be performed; however, this is often not logistically or financially feasible. If patients have had a PET scan before RTP, many insurance companies do not cover a second PET scan. Image registration techniques (fusion) combine data from the PET scan into the separately obtained RTP CT scan. PET fusion to RTP is difficult in HNC because patients are often in a different position (ie, with neck flexed or extended) for RTP CT scans (**Fig. 3**). The most basic technique for fusion is rigid body transformation (rigid fusion), which matches the PET scan with the RTP using only rotational and translational shifts. Another, more sophisticated, fusion method is nonrigid or deformable registration.[20,51] Deformation uses computer algorithms to deform the CT scan that was done in a neutral position to anatomically match the PET/CT image obtained with the patient in a flexed or extended position. There are few reports examining the effect of different PET fusion techniques in HNC,[22] but there is a significant difference between rigid and deformable fusion for head and neck PET scans. One study[52] found that planning tumor volume (PTV) coverage was severely

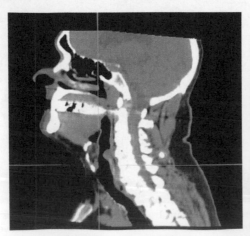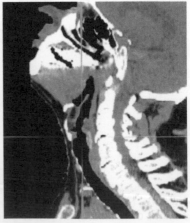

Fig. 3. Difference in neck position between diagnostic CT scan and CT scan for RTP. Diagnostic CT scans are performed in a neutral neck position (*left*), whereas CT scans for RTP are performed in an extended neck position.

compromised using rigid fusion as opposed to deformable fusion; 36.6% of patients in this study would have less than 95% tumor volume coverage with rigid fusion, as opposed to 6.6% of patients with deformable fusion.

Issue 2: Target Definition

One of the areas of controversy in RTP PET scanning is which PET scan volume best represents the gross tumor volume (GTV) and the subsequent PTV.

Multiple methods exist for converting PET data into RTP contours. Several investigators have examined volume differences between CT- and PET-based RTP,[5,53–55] and most studies have shown a decrease in tumor volume when incorporating PET scans. But there is no consensus on how to define PET derived–tumor volumes. Some of the proposed options have been to use manual contouring, an absolute SUV threshold, percentage of SUV maximum, or an automated computer algorithm technique (PET Edge).[5–8,54,55]

Manual contouring is the simplest method to use PET to contour GTV and is based on visual inspection and use of anatomic landmarks. Although this method does not require any image processing or computer software, it has been found to lead to significant interobserver variability.[56]

SUV threshold techniques use a percentage of the maximum SUV (typically 20%–50%) to define the GTV. Threshold techniques can lead to wide volume variation. Ford and colleagues[57] found that the GTV volume can increase by 200% with as little as a 5% change in the SUV threshold level and that a single SUV threshold for all tumors is likely inadequate.[5,7,8]

Absolute SUV techniques use an absolute SUV cutoff (typically 2.5 or 3.0) to define the GTV. This technique is simpler and less arbitrary than the absolute SUV technique because it does not depend on tumor size, and it has been promoted as the optimal way to define HNC GTV by several investigators.[32,58] However, this technique is limited by uncertainty in SUV calculation and in choosing which SUV value to use.

Finally, several automated methods of GTV contouring are available.[6–8,59] These methods use a variety of computer-based algorithms to define the GTV. Most reports using automated techniques have been feasibility studies, with few comparisons[6,59] to clinically defined GTVs or other PET-defined GTVs. Yu and colleagues[9] recently published on a novel automated technique incorporating information from both the PET and CT scans and reported that this automated technique was closer to manually derived volumes than automated threshold SUV or 50% of maximum SUV technique. It is possible that subtle differences in computer algorithms for PET contouring could account for different outcomes and that different algorithms are better suited for different anatomic areas.

There are surprisingly little data on clinical outcomes with different PET contouring methods. Although several investigators have shown differences in tumor volume contouring between methods, there is little clinical correlation.[59] A recent study[59] examined 15 patients with NSCLC who had a PET scan followed by surgical resection. Pathologic tumor size was compared with preoperative PET scan findings. The investigators found that the best correlation between PET and surgical pathology occurred with an SUV threshold of 31% ($\pm$ 11%) and an absolute SUV of 3.0 ($\pm$ 1.6).

A similar study in HNC examined 12 patients who had a PET evaluation of tumor and lymph node size using various PET methods (SUV 2.5, SUV 40%, etc) and compared the PET volumes to the pathologic tumor size. The investigators found that SUV40 had the best correlation with pathologic tumor volume ($R^2 = 0.697$). They also found that SUV40 was more likely to underestimate the tumor volume, whereas SUV2.5 was more likely to overestimate tumor volume.[59] Further studies and larger numbers of patients are needed to validate these results and evaluate different disease sites.

Issue 3: Respiratory Motion

A third issue is that of respiratory motion. Many tumors move with the respiratory cycle; this has been well documented in lung cancer but has also been seen in pancreatic, gastric, esophageal, prostate, and other cancers. Tumor motion obviously has a large effect on radiation therapy delivery, and one of the main purposes of IGRT is to reduce the uncertainty of error from tumor motion, through daily imaging, respiratory gating, or tumor tracking. However, PET scans and thus PET scan–derived contours are also subject to errors from respiratory gating. When a single CT planning image is acquired without breath holding or gating, it captures the anatomy at a random instant in the respiratory cycle. PET is performed over many respiratory cycles and thus provides an image over the whole volume within which the lesion moves. The basic result of this method is that the tumor volume and subsequent SUV are smeared out over the respiratory cycle. The PET image may show an apparent increase in the lesion size and a decrease in the SUV. Phantom studies have shown that in the case of a moving object rather than for a static one, a lower threshold should be used for an accurate assessment of its volume.[60–62] One obvious solution to this is to have a gated PET-CT scan acquisition. This technology results in more accurate PET volumes than a nongated PET scan. Such precision can be especially valuable when high-dose radiosurgery for lung lesions is being used. When nongated PET scans are used, target volume definition should take tumor motion into account, and the threshold level should be carefully chosen when automated methods are used. One potential benefit of the nongated PET scan is that it may have the capability of demonstrating the degree of motion of the tumor; in essence, it can act as a poor man's 4-dimensional (4D) CT. However, it is unclear if the tumor motion that would be demonstrated with a dedicated 4D CT scan is the same as the low dose effect of the nongated PET scan, and caution is urged.

SUMMARY

PET scans are becoming increasingly important in oncology. PET scans are well established in staging and follow-up for several cancers, and there is active exploration into using PET scans as a prognostic and perhaps even a predictive tool. In addition, PET scans also have a special use in RTP. PET scans allow for better target definition, which is increasingly important as the technology used to deliver radiation improves. PET scans have several areas that remain controversial including the optimal way to define gross tumor via PET (ie, using SUV threshold, SUV percentage of maximum, or PET algorithm tool), how to incorporate PET scans not obtained in the radiation therapy treatment position, and how to account for respiratory motion in PET scans.

REFERENCES

1. Warburg O, Posener K, Negelein E. Uber den stoffwechsel der carcinomzelle. Biochem Z 1924;152: 309–35 [in German].
2. Keyes JW Jr. SUV: standard uptake or silly useless value? J Nucl Med 1995;36(10):1836–9.
3. Frank SJ, Chao KS, Schwartz DL, et al. Technology insight: PET and PET/CT in head and neck tumor staging and radiation therapy planning. Nat Clin Pract Oncol 2005;2(10):526–33.
4. Giraud P, Grahek D, Montravers F, et al. CT and 18F-deoxyglucose (FDG) image fusion for optimization of conformal radiotherapy of lung cancers. Int J Radiat Oncol Biol Phys 2001;49:1249–57.
5. Paulino AC, Koshy M, Howell R, et al. Comparison of CT- and FDG-PET-defined gross tumor volume in intensity-modulated radiotherapy for head-and-neck cancer. Int J Radiat Oncol Biol Phys 2005;61: 1385–92.
6. Greco C, Nehmeh SA, Schöder H, et al. Evaluation of different methods of 18F-FDG-PET target volume delineation in the radiotherapy of head and neck cancer. Am J Clin Oncol 2008;31(5): 439–45.
7. El-Bassiouni M, Ciernik IF, Davis JB, et al. [18FDG] PET-CT-based intensity-modulated radiotherapy treatment planning of head and neck cancer. Int J Radiat Oncol Biol Phys 2007;69(1):286–93.
8. Geets X, Lee JA, Bol A, et al. A gradient-based method for segmenting FDG-PET images: methodology and validation. Eur J Nucl Med Mol Imaging 2007;34(9):1427–38.
9. Yu H, Caldwell C, Mah K, et al. Automated radiation targeting in head-and-neck cancer using region-based texture analysis of PET and CT images. Int J Radiat Oncol Biol Phys 2009;75(2):618–25.
10. Yu J, Li X, Xing L, et al. Comparison of tumor volumes as determined by pathologic examination and FDG-PET/CT images of non-small-cell lung cancer: a pilot study. Int J Radiat Oncol Biol Phys 2009;75(5):1468–74.
11. Hunt MA, Zelefsky MJ, Wolden S, et al. Treatment planning and delivery of intensity-modulated radiation therapy for primary nasopharynx cancer. Int J Radiat Oncol Biol Phys 2001;49:623–32.
12. Kam MK, Chau RM, Suen J, et al. Intensity-modulated radiotherapy in nasopharyngeal carcinoma: dosimetric advantage over conventional plans and feasibility of dose escalation. Int J Radiat Oncol Biol Phys 2003;56:145–57.
13. Den RB, Doemer A, Kubicek G, et al. Daily image guidance with cone-beam computed tomography for head-and-neck cancer intensity-modulated radiotherapy: a prospective study. Int J Radiat Oncol Biol Phys 2010;76(5):1353–9.
14. Ido T, Wan CN, Casella V, et al. Labeled 2-dexoy-D-glucose analogs: 18F labeled 2-deoxy-2-fluoro-D-glucose, 2-deoxy-2-fluoro-D-mannose and 14C-2-deoxy-2-fluoro-D-glucose. J Labelled Comp Radiopharm 1978;14:175–83.
15. Trautmann TG, Zuger JH. Positron emission tomography for pretreatment staging and post-treatment evaluation in cancer of the anal canal. Mol Imaging Biol 2005;7:309–13.
16. Cotter SE, Gigsby PW, Siegel BA, et al. FDG-PET/CT in the evaluation of anal carcinoma. Int J Radiat Oncol Biol Phys 2006;65:720–5.
17. Winton E, Heriot AG, Ng M, et al. The impact of 18-FDG positron emission tomography on the staging, management and outcome of anal cancer. Br J Cancer 2009;100:693–700.

18. Gould MK, Maclean CC, Kuschner WG, et al. Accuracy of positron emission tomography for diagnosis of pulmonary nodules and mass lesions: a meta-analysis. JAMA 2001;285:914–24.

19. Gould MK, Kuschner WG, Rydzak CE, et al. Test performance of positron emission tomography and computed tomography for mediastinal staging in patients with non-small-cell lung cancer: a meta-analysis. Ann Intern Med 2003;139:879–92.

20. Shreve PD, Anzai Y, Wahl RL. Pitfalls in oncologic diagnosis with FDG PET imaging: physiologic and benign variants. Radiographics 1999;19:61–77.

21. Bakheet SM, Powe J. Fluorine-18-fluorodeoxyglucose uptake in rheumatoid arthritis-associated lung disease in a patient with thyroid cancer. J Nucl Med 1998;39:234–6.

22. Bakheet SM, Powe J, Kandil A, et al. F-18 FDG uptake in breast infection and inflammation. Clin Nucl Med 2000;25:100–3.

23. Bakheet SM, Saleem M, Powe J, et al. F-18 fluorodeoxyglucose chest uptake in lung inflammation and infection. Clin Nucl Med 2000;25:273–8.

24. Kubicek G, Fogh S, Piper JW, et al. PET registration methods and dosimetric consequences. Int J Radiat Oncol Biol Phys 2009;75(3 Suppl):S74–5.

25. Koike I, Ohmura M, Hata M, et al. FDG-PET scanning alter radiation can predict tumor regrowth three months later. Int J Radiat Oncol Biol Phys 2003;57: 1231–8.

26. Pieterman RM, Que TH, Elsinga PH, et al. Comparison of (11)C-choline and (18)F-FDG PET in primary diagnosis and staging of patients with thoracic cancer. J Nucl Med 2002;43:167–72.

27. Pieterman RM, van Putten JW, Meuzelaar JJ, et al. Preoperative staging of non-small cell lung cancer with positron-emission tomography. N Engl J Med 2000;343:254–61.

28. Hutchings M, Mikhaeel NG, Fields PA, et al. Prognostic value of interim FDG-PET after two or three cycles of chemotherapy in Hodgkin lymphoma. Ann Oncol 2005;16:1160–8.

29. Choi JY, Lee KH, Shim YM, et al. Improved detection of individual nodal involvement in squamous cell carcinoma of the esophagus by FDG PET. J Nucl Med 2000;41:808–15.

30. Bradley J, Thorstad WL, Mutic S, et al. Impact of FDG-PET on radiation therapy volume delineation in non-small-cell lung cancer. Int J Radiat Oncol Biol Phys 2004;59:78–86.

31. Ciernik IF, Dizendorf E, Baumert BG, et al. Radiation treatment planning with an integrated positron emission and computer tomography (PET/CT): a feasibility study. Int J Radiat Oncol Biol Phys 2003;57(3):853–63.

32. Wang D, Schultz CJ, Jursinic PA, et al. Initial experience of FDG-PET/CT guided IMRT of head-and-neck carcinoma. Int J Radiat Oncol Biol Phys 2006;65:143–51.

33. Heron DE, Andrade RS, Beriwal S, et al. PET-CT in radiation oncology: the impact on diagnosis, treatment planning, and assessment of treatment response. Am J Clin Oncol 2008;31(4):352–62.

34. Heron DE, Smith RP, Andrade RS. Advances in image-guided radiation therapy–the role of PET-CT. Med Dosim 2006;31(1):3–11.

35. Geets X, Daisne JF, Tomsej M, et al. Impact of the type of imaging modality on target volumes delineation and dose distribution in pharyngo- laryngeal squamous cell carcinoma: comparison between pre- and per-treatment studies. Radiother Oncol 2006;78:291–7.

36. Daisne JF, Duprez T, Weynand B, et al. Tumor volume in pharyngolaryngeal squamous cell carcinoma: comparison at CT, MR imaging, and FDG PET and validation with surgical specimen. Radiology 2004;233:93–100.

37. Vernon MR, Maheshwari M, Schultz CJ, et al. Clinical outcomes of patients receiving integrated PET/CT-guided radiotherapy for head and neck carcinoma. Int J Radiat Oncol Biol Phys 2008;70: 678–84.

38. Paulino AC, Johnstone PA. FDG-PET in radiotherapy treatment planning: Pandora's box? Int J Radiat Oncol Biol Phys 2004;59:4–5.

39. Lucignani G, Jereczek-Fossa BA, Orecchia R. The role of molecular imaging in precision radiation therapy for target definition, treatment planning optimization and quality control. Eur J Nucl Med Mol Imaging 2004;31:1059–63.

40. Leong T, Everitt C, Yuen K, et al. A prospective study to evaluate the impact of FDG-PET on CT-based radiotherapy treatment planning for oesophageal cancer. Radiother Oncol 2006;78:254–61.

41. Moureau-Zabotto L, Touboul E, Lerouge D, et al. Impact of CT and 18Fdeoxyglucose positron emission tomography image fusion for conformal radiotherapy in esophageal carcinoma. Int J Radiat Oncol Biol Phys 2005;63:340–5.

42. Anderson C, Koshy M, Staley C, et al. PET-CT fusion in radiation management of patients with anorectal tumors. Int J Radiat Oncol Biol Phys 2007;69:155–62.

43. Nguyen BT, Joon DL, Khoo V, et al. Assessing the impact of FDG-PET in the management of anal cancer. Radiother Oncol 2008;87:376–82.

44. Narayan K, Hicks RJ, Jobling T, et al. A comparison of MRI and PET scanning in surgically staged locoregionally advanced cervical cancer: potential impact on treatment. Int J Gynecol Cancer 2001; 11:263–71.

45. Khan N, Oriuchi N, Yoshizaki A, et al. Diagnostic accuracy of FDG PET imaging for the detection of recurrent or metastatic gynecologic cancer. Ann Nucl Med 2005;19:137–45.

46. Grisaru D, Almog B, Levine C, et al. The diagnostic accuracy of 18Ffluorodeoxyglucose PET/CT in

patients with gynecological malignancies. Gynecol Oncol 2004;94:680–4.

47. Nakamoto Y, Saga T, Fujii S. Positron emission tomography application for gynecologic tumors. Int J Gynecol Cancer 2005;15:701–9.

48. Esthappan J, Mutic S, Malyapa RS, et al. Treatment planning guidelines regarding the use of CT/PET-guided IMRT for cervical carcinoma with positive paraaortic lymph nodes. Int J Radiat Oncol Biol Phys 2004;58:1289–97.

49. Mutic S, Malyapa RS, Grigsby PW, et al. PET-guided IMRT for cervical carcinoma with positive para-aortic lymph nodes—a dose-escalation treatment planning study. Int J Radiat Oncol Biol Phys 2003;55:28–35.

50. Mutic S, Grigsby PW, Low DA, et al. PET-guided three-dimensional treatment planning of intracavitary gynecologic implants. Int J Radiat Oncol Biol Phys 2002;52:1104–10.

51. Sweet WH. The use of nuclear disintegration in diagnosis and treatment of brain tumors. N Engl J Med 1951;245:875–8.

52. Kubicek GJ, Champ C, Fogh S, et al. FDG-PET staging and importance of lymph node SUV in head and neck cancer. Head Neck Oncol 2010;2:19.

53. Heron DE, Andrade RS, Flickinger J, et al. Hybrid PET-CT simulation for radiation treatment planning in head-and-neck cancers: a brief technical report. Int J Radiat Oncol Biol Phys 20041;60(5):1419–24.

54. Schinagl DA, Vogel WV, Hoffmann AL, et al. Comparison of five segmentation tools for 18F-fluoro-deoxy-glucose-positron emission tomography-based target volume definition in head and neck cancer. Int J Radiat Oncol Biol Phys 2007;69(4):1282–9.

55. Scarfone C, Lavely WC, Cmelak AJ, et al. Prospective feasibility trial of radiotherapy target definition for head and neck cancer using 3-dimensional PET and CT imaging. J Nucl Med 2004;45(4):543–52.

56. Riegel AC, Berson AM, Destian S, et al. Variability of gross tumor volume delineation in head-and-neck cancer using CT and PET/CT fusion. Int J Radiat Oncol Biol Phys 2006;65(3):726–32.

57. Ford EC, Kinahan PE, Hanlon L, et al. Tumor delineation using PET in head and neck cancers: threshold contouring and lesion volumes. Med Phys 2006; 33(11):4280–8.

58. Daisne JF, Sibomana M, Bol A, et al. Evaluation of a multimodality image (CT, MRI and PET) coregistration procedure on phantom and head and neck cancer patients: accuracy, reproducibility and consistency. Radiother Oncol 2003;69(3):237–45.

59. Burri RJ, Rangaswamy B, Kostakoglu L, et al. Correlation of positron emission tomography standard uptake value and pathologic specimen size in cancer of the head and neck. Int J Radiat Oncol Biol Phys 2008;71(3):682–8.

60. Yaremko B, Riauka T, Robinson D, et al. Thresholding in PET images of static and moving targets. Phys Med Biol 2005;50:5969–82.

61. Yaremko B, Riauka T, Robinson D, et al. Threshold modification for tumour imaging in non-small-cell lung cancer using positron emission tomography. Nucl Med Commun 2005;26:433–40.

62. Lodge MA, Badawi RD, Gilbert R, et al. Comparison of 2- dimensional and 3-dimensional acquisition for 18F-FDG PET oncology studies performed on an LSO-based scanner. J Nucl Med 2006;47: 23–31.

63. Roh JL, Ryu CH, Kim JS, et al. Utility of 2-[^{18}F] fluoro-2-deoxy-D-glucose positron emission tomography and positron emission tomography/computed tomography imaging in the preoperative staging of head and neck squamous cell carcinoma. Oral Oncol 2007;43(9):887–93.

64. Kubicek GJ, Kimler BF, Reddy EK, et al. PET scans for staging and follow-up for head and neck cancers treated with radiotherapy. Oral presentation Radiographic Society of North American (RSNA) 2007 annual meeting. Abstract # 6001178.

65. Schwartz DL, Rajendran J, Yueh B, et al. FDG-PET prediction of head and neck squamous cell cancer outcomes. Arch Otolaryngol Head Neck Surg 2004;130(12):1361–7.

66. Allal AS, Slosman DO, Kebdani T, et al. Prediction of outcome in head-and-neck cancer patients using the standardized uptake value of 2-[18F]fluoro-2-deoxy-D-glucose. Int J Radiat Oncol Biol Phys 2004;59(5):1295–300.

67. Kitagawa Y, Nishizawa S, Sano K, et al. Prospective comparison of 18F-FDG PET with conventional imaging modalities (MRI, CT, and 67Ga scintigraphy) in assessment of combined intraarterial chemotherapy and radiotherapy for head and neck carcinoma. J Nucl Med 2003;44(2):198–206.

68. Halfpenny W, Hain SF, Biassoni L, et al. FDG-PET. A possible prognostic factor in head and neck cancer. Br J Cancer 2002;86(4):512–6.

69. Brun E, Kjellén E, Tennvall J, et al. FDG PET studies during treatment: prediction of therapy outcome in head and neck squamous cell carcinoma. Head Neck 2002;24(2):127–35.

70. Greven KM, Williams DW 3rd, McGuirt WF Sr, et al. Serial positron emission tomography scans following radiation therapy of patients with head and neck cancer. Head Neck 2001;23(11):942–6.

71. Minn H, Lapela M, Klemi PJ, et al. Prediction of survival with fluorine-18-fluoro-deoxyglucose and PET in head and neck cancer. J Nucl Med 1997; 38(12):1907–11.

72. van Baardwijk A, Dooms C, van Suylen RJ, et al. The maximum uptake of (18)F-deoxyglucose on positron emission tomography scan correlates with survival, hypoxia inducible factor-1alpha and GLUT-1 in

non-small cell lung cancer. Eur J Cancer 2007;43(9): 1392–8.

73. Vesselle H, Salskov A, Turcotte E, et al. Relationship between non-small cell lung cancer FDG uptake at PET, tumor histology, and Ki-67 proliferation index. J Thorac Oncol 2008;3(9):971–8.

74. Cerfolio RJ, Bryant AS, Winokur TS, et al. Repeat FDG-PET after neoadjuvant therapy is a predictor of pathologic response in patients with non-small cell lung cancer. Ann Thorac Surg 2004;78(6):1903–9.

75. Downey RJ, Akhurst T, Gonen M, et al. Preoperative F-18 fluorodeoxyglucose-positron emission tomography maximal standardized uptake value predicts survival after lung cancer resection. J Clin Oncol 2004;22(16):3255–60.

76. Jeong HJ, Min JJ, Park JM, et al. Determination of the prognostic value of [(18)F]fluorodeoxyglucose uptake by using positron emission tomography in patients with non-small cell lung cancer. Nucl Med Commun 2002;23(9):865–70.

77. Higashi K, Ueda Y, Arisaka Y, et al. 18F-FDG uptake as a biologic prognostic factor for recurrence in patients with surgically resected non-small cell lung cancer. J Nucl Med 2002;43(1):39–45.

78. Vanuytsel LJ, Vansteenkiste JF, Stroobants SG, et al. Prognostic importance of the standardized uptake value on (18)F-fluoro-2-deoxy-glucose-positron emission tomography scan in non-small-cell lung cancer: an analysis of 125 cases. Leuven Lung Cancer Group. J Clin Oncol 1999;17(10): 3201–6.

79. Okereke IC, Gangadharan SP, Kent MS, et al. Standard uptake value predicts survival in non-small cell lung cancer. Ann Thorac Surg 2009;88(3):911–5.

Technical Aspects of PET/CT-Based Radiotherapy Planning

Tim Fox, PhD[a],*, Josh Lawson, MD[b],
Eduard Schreibmann, PhD[a]

KEYWORDS

- Image registration • Segmentation • PET • CT

Incorporation of information from more than one image study into another image study is encouraged by the desire to use the most complete information available for improved decision making. Color-enhanced imagery from satellite data is a method meteorologists use to aid them with satellite interpretation. The combination of geographical information (map) and satellite imagery has enhanced value to the meteorologist using image fusion techniques as opposed to interpreting the information separately.

Physicians have understood the importance of fusing information from multiple images for developing a comprehensive diagnostic overview of the patient.[1,2] This practice has become even more significant with the growing number of tomographic imaging methods. PET/computed tomography (CT) has been used for both diagnosis/staging of cancer and guiding the cancer treatment planning process. PET-guided radiotherapy (RT) planning has been increasingly used to assist in determining the exact tumor locations so that therapy procedures can be focused on the tumor, minimizing damage to the surrounding tissue. However, incorporating PET/CT into the treatment planning process raises challenges in areas of immobilization, image registration, and target volume segmentation. This article focuses on the technical aspects of integrating PET/CT into RT

planning and presents a general overview of the clinical workflow and challenges involved in the planning.

RADIOTHERAPY IMAGING SYSTEMS
CT Simulation

Over the past decade, many radiation oncology departments have incorporated the modern CT simulator into their treatment process, alleviating the need to use a conventional x-ray simulator. Commercial CT simulators that provide 3-dimensional (3D) volumetric RT techniques are available to be used on a routine basis in clinical departments.[3–10] CT simulation combines some of the functions of an image-based, 3D treatment planning system and conventional simulator. A CT simulator software system recreates the treatment machine and allows import, manipulation, display, and storage of images from CT. The CT simulation scanner table must have a flat top similar to that of RT treatment machines. Besides the flat tabletop, CT scanners used for CT simulation are usually equipped with external patient marking/positioning lasers that can be fixed or mobile.

PET and PET/CT

PET is a molecular imaging modality capable of detecting small concentrations of positron-emitting

a Department of Radiation Oncology, Emory University School of Medicine, 1365 Clifton Road, Atlanta, GA 30322, USA
b Department of Radiation Oncology, University of California, 3855 Health Sciences Drive, San Diego, CA 92103, USA
* Corresponding author.
E-mail address: tim@radonc.emory.org

PET Clin 6 (2011) 117–129
doi:10.1016/j.cpet.2011.02.005

radioisotopes. Most PET scanners use curved tabletops as opposed to flat tabletops for CT simulation and RT, causing some difficulty in registering PET and CT data sets, depending on the patient's position at the time of the imaging scans. The first combined PET/CT scanner was developed to provide an automated hardware solution to the need for coregistered anatomic and functional images.[11] An accurate and precise rigid transformation for coregistering the CT and PET images is determined by carefully aligning the 2 scanners during installation and measuring their physical offset. This method eliminates one of the major limitations of software registration approaches by providing a constant spatial transformation between PET and CT images that is known beforehand and is independent of patient positioning. The underlying assumption is that the patient does not move during the procedure. The accuracy of software-based registration methods is typically on the order of the voxel size of the modality with the lowest spatial resolution.[12] In the case of PET and CT coregistration, this accuracy typically corresponds to 4 to 5 mm. In contrast, the intrinsic registration accuracy of a combined PET-CT scanner is submillimeter.

4D CT and 4D PET/CT

A new method of CT simulation is known as 4-dimensional (4D) CT simulation (3D + time = 4D). In one method of 4D CT simulation, retrospective gating of the CT simulation data is performed using the patient's breathing cycle.[13] GE Medical Systems (Milwaukee, WS, USA) and Varian Medical Systems (Palo Alto, CA, USA) have developed a system using the RPM Respiratory Gating system with a multislice CT scanner for analyzing and incorporating intrafraction motion management using tomographic data sets. The system provides retrospective gating of the tomographic data set by taking 3D data sets at specific time intervals to create a time-dependent 4D CT imaging study.[13] The use of this 4D imaging set allows the physician to accurately define the target and its trajectory with respect to normal anatomy and critical structures. This type of CT simulation tool can then be used with the respiratory gating system at the treatment machine to gate the beam delivery with the patient's breathing cycle. The use of 4D CT simulation makes it possible to acquire CT scans that provide new information on the motion of tumors and critical structures. PET gating has been performed with a camera-based patient monitoring system and has shown a volume reduction of tumors by as much as 34%.[14] The same method of patient monitoring has also been used to perform gated RT of liver tumors.[15] Respiratory gating is now available for 4D PET/CT.

INTEGRATING PET/CT IMAGING INTO RT PLANNING

The PET image data must be accurately and efficiently integrated into the treatment cycle of the patient undergoing RT. For external beam RT, the patient treatment cycle consists of simulation, planning, delivery, and verification. Three possible scenarios for integrating PET/CT into the RT planning process are presented in the following sections.

Scenario 1: PET/CT Simulation

The first scenario is the simplest, in which a PET/CT simulator is used for CT simulation of the treatment planning process. The patient is placed in the PET/CT scanner using their immobilization device that provides for reproducible positioning during treatment delivery. The PET/CT scanner is equipped with a laser marking system, and the patient's tumor location is marked on the skin for reference. In this situation, there is no need to register via software another imaging data set to the CT simulation; the dual-scanner system uses the automatic physical registration for this process. This scenario ensures that the patient is in the treatment position for both the PET and CT scans. However, for many radiation oncology centers, the use of PET/CT simulation requires the additional expense of a dedicated PET/CT for radiation oncology purposes.

Scenario 2: CT Simulation Followed by PET/CT Procedure

The patient is scanned in the CT simulator using a custom immobilization device to acquire the treatment planning CT data set. Following CT simulation, the patient is scanned in a PET/CT scanner along with their custom-made immobilization system for the imaging procedure. After the scan, the PET/CT data set is registered with the planning CT data set, using various methods described in a later section. The registration is typically CT to CT to determine the coordinate system transformation. Once this CT-CT transformation is computed, the PET images are registered with the planning CT images for functional target delineation.

Scenario 3: Diagnostic PET/CT Procedure Followed by CT Simulation

The patient receives a diagnostic PET/CT procedure before the CT simulation procedure, which is performed using diagnostic imaging protocols such as curved tabletops and different patient positioning. A custom immobilization device is created, and the CT simulation procedure is performed to acquire the treatment planning CT data set. The PET/CT images are then registered to the planning CT images. With this scenario, accuracy of image registration is difficult to achieve because the patient was likely scanned in a different position between the 2 systems. This scenario is not ideal because many rigid image registration methods fail to register the images correctly. Deformable or nonrigid image registration methods may be more appropriate to match the PET/CT images to the planning CT images.

Of the 3 scenarios, the second and third have challenges that limit the accuracy of the image registration algorithms for multimodal images. One problem is the degree of similarity of the patient's position and shape during the image acquisitions. The other issue is the differences in time when acquiring the image data sets. When performing scans in the thorax and abdominal region, motion artifacts present a problem when registering PET/CT images with planning CT images. The use of deformable image registration methods may help overcome these challenges. The use of 4D PET/CT may address the motion artifacts encountered by respiration. At present, scenarios 1 and 2 are recommended for clinical environment because it is important to image the patient in the treatment immobilization devices for accurate image registration.

IMAGE REGISTRATION METHODS

Registration is the process of matching 2 images based on their content. With the advent of different imaging modalities, it is common to have various data sets of the same anatomy acquired on different scanners. The patient is usually aligned to the scanner's coordinate system by lasers or other positioning devices, but the patient may have different postures in the scans. A procedure to match the image studies based on the information within the images as opposed to external references is required to compare and correlate the information within the scans. This matching can be either manual, whereby an operator manipulates one image to match its information to another, or automated, whereby the computer finds the optimal transformation by an optimization procedure.

Many image registration methods have been implemented based on either the geometrical features (pointlike anatomic features or surfaces)[9,16–20] or intensity similarity measures

(mutual information [MI]).[21,22] Registration establishes an exact point-to-point correspondence (coordinate system transformation) between the voxels of the different modalities, making direct comparison possible. Transformations are either rigid or nonrigid (sometimes called curved, deformable, or elastic). A rigid coordinate transformation is when only translations in 3 orthogonal directions and rotations in 3 directions are allowed. Nonrigid transformations are more complex, with nonlinear scaling or warping of 1 data set as well as rotation and translations. The image registration procedure is a 3-step process:

1. Identify relevant features in both volumes to be matched (with some methods using segmentation or classification).
2. Define a similarity metric (cost function) to measure how well 2 images are aligned.
3. Search for the best transformation to bring the 2 images into spatial alignment.

The image that is being matched is typically called the fixed or target image. The image that is moving its coordinate system to match the fixed image is called the moving or floating image. The organization of image registration methods in the literature can be based on the nature of the matching base or transformation. According to the nature of the matching base, medical image registration is divided into 4 main categories: manual, landmark based, surface based, and volume based. In this section, the image registration methods are described for 3D/3D registration of 2 images, in which all dimensions are spatial. In some instances, the dimension of time may be added to the registration process. However, the following descriptions are for 3D/3D registration, which applies to 2 tomographic data sets. A brief description of rigid and deformable registration methods is provided in this section.

Rigid Registration

Manual or interactive registration
Interactive or manual methods allow physicians to gain complete control over the registration process. Image data sets may be translated and rotated with respect to the fixed image data set.[23] The translation and rotations create the coordinate transformation between the 2 image data sets. Some image registration framework provides fast reformatting of sagittal and coronal slices to give immediate feedback of rigid body transformations to the physician by fusing the 2 image data sets. Interactive registration methods commonly suffer from a subjective validation of the registration processes. However, automated

volume-based registration methods also use a subjective validation process to review the registration results. The accuracy of registration depends on the user's judgment on the correlation between anatomic features. The main advantages of manual methods are intuitive handling, immediate display of results, and that time is not consumed preprocessing. The disadvantages are poor reproducibility and no metric indicating the goodness of the registration.

Landmark-based registration
Landmark registration uses corresponding points located within different images to determine the spatial transformation between the paired points.[20,24–26] Landmark-based registration methods can be divided into 2 types: external landmarks and internal landmarks. External landmarks are based on foreign objects introduced into the images, such as a stereotactic frame attached to the patient for brain imaging. These external markers need to be visible on all image sets. This marker may be metal for CT images and Gallium-68 for PET imaging. External methods rely on objects attached to the patient, which are visible in all the imaging modalities. Because the markers can be easily seen in the imaging modalities, the image registration algorithms can be automated and sped up without the need for a complex optimization algorithm. One of the disadvantages of external landmarks is that the placement of the markers usually requires an invasive procedure. Internal landmarks, referred to as anatomic markers, are points of internal anatomy that can be visualized or located within each image. A physician or clinical expert using an interactive software method of locating the points on both image sets identifies these internal markers. After identifying the landmarks, the image registration algorithm calculates the geometrical transformation by minimizing a cost function representing the mismatch between the image sets. This cost function may be the distance between the coordinates of these landmarks. Landmark-based methods are mostly used to find rigid transformations, and the set of identified points is sparse compared with that of volume-based intensity methods, which allows for relatively fast optimization procedures. The identification of internal anatomic points is a segmentation procedure and involves locating 4 to 10 points on corresponding sets of images. When registering PET images to CT images, common anatomic points can be difficult to locate even for the medical expert. In addition, the spatial resolution of PET imaging makes the use of internal landmarks difficult to apply to nuclear medicine imaging.

Volume-based registration
Multimodal imaging, such as PET/CT, MR/CT, and PET/MR, pose difficulty when image registration is used, and is difficult to achieve with landmark-based methods because it is difficult to identify or segment common structures in both image sets. Over the past 15 years, automated image registration methods have increasingly used volume or intensity-based matching algorithms.[1,21,22] Volume-based image registration methods are different from others because they operate directly with the image intensity (gray values) values without user interaction. The volume-based methods for 3D/3D image registration require large computational costs that have become available over the past decade to enable these methods in routine clinical practice. The most common volume-based image registration method uses the full image content and intensity values for the registration process. Intensity-based registration methods measure the similarity of 2 images by the statistical description and optimize it by adjusting the transformation parameters. The simplest similarity measures are those that directly compare intensity values between the 2 images, voxel by voxel. However, this measure is only appropriate for monomodal image fusion, such as CT to CT. For multimodal image registration, other measures are needed because there is a different assignment of intensity values to various tissues. For example, bone is bright in CT and dark in MR imaging, whereas air is dark in both MR and CT. Thus, other similarity measures are needed for multimodal image registration, such as minimum variance or MI. The minimum variance measure is based on the concept that an image consists of largely uniform regions that differ substantially (large variance) from one another. If the 2 images are correctly registered, a uniform region in 1 image corresponds to a uniform region in the other image, even though the mean intensity values are unrelated.

A popular similarity measure using the voxel intensity histogram for multimodal image registration is the MI method. The use of MI for medical image registration applications was independently introduced in 1995 by Maes and colleagues[21] and Wells and colleagues.[22] This method is based on the assumption that there is a correlation between groups of voxels that have similar values. MI measures how much information one random variable (image intensity in one image) reveals about another (image intensity in the other image). For 2 images, the MI is computed from the joint probability distribution of the images' pixel intensity values. When 2 images are aligned, the joint probability distribution is a sharp peak resulting in a high MI value. An automated MI algorithm searches for a transformation between the fixed and the moving images, at which identical anatomic landmarks of both images are most closely overlapping. A general optimizer seeks the global maximum of a cost value (provided by the cost function) by iteratively modifying the parameters according to the optimization scheme. The similarity measure based on MI is used to compare the pixel intensities in the fixed image, $I_{fixed}(i, j, k)$, with the pixel intensities in the moving image, $I_{moving}(i, j, k)$, where (i, j, k) defines the position of a voxel of the fixed or moving image. The optimizer's task is to find the global maximum of the similarity measure between the 2 images within the search space. In multimodal registration, the MI technique has become a standard reference in medical imaging with the implementation in commercial treatment planning systems. The implementation of MI in clinical practice usually combines interactive manual matching with automated MI image registration. The user uses the interactive mode to manually align the 2 image sets with a close approximation and then applies the automated MI method for final matching of the 2 image sets. This method helps improve the probability of success for MI because it works best when there are no large rotations or translations between the data sets.

Deformable Registration

The image registration methods presented thus far have assumed that the 2 image sets could be registered using rigid registration. However, this is not always the case because the patient can be positioned differently between imaging scans and the internal organs can change position and shape. This change may be because of respiration for the lungs and degree of filling for the bladder. Deformable or elastic registration methods can be used for these situations, but they present additional challenges. An active area of image registration research addresses the deformable image registration methods.[27–30]

As opposed to rigid registration, deformable registration is able to account for local changes such as displacement and deformation of soft internal organs, further increasing accuracy of the treatment planning process. Rigid registration typically considers only the 6 parameters that are optimized to correlate the fixed and moving images, but deformable registration defines a displacement vector for each voxel in the input

images to model fine changes within the patient or between scans. Although the aim of deformable image registration is straightforward, a simple optimization procedure cannot reliably solve the problem of finding a deformation field that closely matches a target image to a reference image. The deformation field is in essence a matrix of displacement vectors for each voxel location. Displacement vectors' magnitude is unknown but can be obtained by minimizing the differences between the deformed template and the original reference image. This optimization problem can be solved by different optimization methods spanning a trade-off between speed and accuracy by making different assumptions to constrain the number of solutions and reduce the search space by focusing on specific features within the image or by placing restrictions on the deformation field. Vectors are not treated separately, which ensures that the displacement field correctly simulates the underlying anatomic changes, with almost all algorithms using a regularization term to force smoothness of the displacement field.

Standard registration algorithms consist of the following components:

- Metric, defining in mathematical terms what a good match is
- Transform, defining the allowable mapping between the input images
- Optimizer, searching for the transform parameters that minimize the metric.

Technically, the metric quantitatively describes the degree or quality of matching. The optimization algorithm just searches for the transform parameters that minimize the metric value. By the nature of this transform, the algorithms can be categorized into rigid, affine, and deformable. As discussed earlier, a rigid transformation corrects changes in patient posture through translations and rotations. An affine transform also considers possible shear occurring in the patient anatomy between scans. The most accurate mapping is provided when a deformable transform is used, as displacements in every voxel are considered. However, this comes at increased computational demands because a transform defining a deformable mapping is composed of many variables. Indeed, although standard rigid transforms consider only 6 variables (3 translations and 3 rotations), the number of variables to be optimized reaches thousands even for models using interpolations such as the BSpline transform. This model simplifies the problem by superimposing on the images a grid of virtual nodes. Only displacements in these grid nodes are considered in the optimization, with spline functions used to interpolate displacements at an arbitrary location inside the nodes.

The metric or cost function defines what a good deformation is by reproducing the sometimes unclear clinical concepts through equations to quantify the quality of a displacement field. For example, when manually matching 2 data sets, the operator translates one data set to match similar features such as anatomic markers or internal organs shapes. If the operator's judgment can be described in mathematical terms, automatic methods can be used to reproduce his or her actions. When matching internal organs, the operator minimizes differences in image intensities between the 2 images; this is described in mathematical terms by just minimizing differences in voxel intensities. When images are acquired on different modalities, with organs displayed with different intensity levels, more sophisticated cost functions that minimize statistical differences are used, with the MI being the most popular. The best deformation field has displacements that minimize the cost function. These optimal values are found in an optimization procedure that iteratively modifies displacements and calculates the corresponding cost function, also obtaining feedback on needed displacement changes that would further minimize the cost function. Although any general-purpose optimization approach can be used to find the best correlation, gradient-based algorithms are by far preferred for their convergence speed. Because of its significant improvements in targeting accuracy, and with different vendors offering deformable registration algorithms as part of their software solutions, clinicians may use the procedure soon as part of their standard treatment practice.

Validation of Image Registration Methods

Image registration provides an approximate solution to the problem of matching the 2 imaging data sets. The use of rigid or deformable registration may improve the solution, but the clinician should always realize that image registration is an approximation. The quality assurance of image registration methods is difficult to perform for all automated systems because the ground truth for each patient is unknown. The ideal image registration method would provide an uncertainty value on the accuracy of the image registration. This uncertainty could then be incorporated into the radiation treatment planning process by adding margins to the registered functional image structures, which would indicate the spatial uncertainty of the image match. Landmark-based image registration methods can provide a measure of the accuracy of the result.[31] For example, the mean squared distances between the matched anatomic points can be computed to give an estimate of the image registration accuracy. However, there is unknown uncertainty in the identification of the points, which cannot be quantitatively represented. Grosu and colleagues[32] described a procedure for validating a commercial MI image registration method using PET and CT images of the brain. A relocatable head mask along with a stereotactic imaging localizer was used for both PET and CT images. Reference markers were placed on the stereotactic localizer and were visible in PET and CT images; this system was referred to as the gold standard. Thus, the investigators used an external frame system to evaluate the accuracy of the automated MI image registration method. In this study, a mean deviation of the MI-based automatic CT/PET fusion compared with the external marker–based fusion was 2.4 ± 0.54 mm. Considering the PET resolution of about 3 to 4 mm and the possibility of error in the fusion (2.4 mm), the investigators recommend a safety margin of approximately 3 mm for the functional target volumes.[32]

Careful case-by-case inspection of algorithm accuracy in describing anatomic changes is essential to assure safe and accurate practice of RT, with a quality assurance protocol ideally identifying regions where the deformation field is unrealistic and using qualitative rather than quantitative evaluation measures. As opposed to rigid registration, in which only one valid solution is attainable, deformable registration problems do not have a unique solution, making algorithm verification problematic. Early reports of the deformable registration technology estimated accuracy by using concepts developed for rigid registration,[33–40] such as using markers or visible anatomic landmarks to assess accuracy of a deformable registration solution. This method is tedious, as between 36 and 1050 landmarks were reported to be needed to achieve an accuracy with a 95% confidence interval within a 0.5-mm range,[41] and provides misleading results, as the method does not provide any measure of accuracy inside structures of uniform contrast[42] or far away from the markers. Specialized approaches that target specific applications of a deformable registration algorithm have been proposed recently. For example, a valid approach if the deformation algorithm is used for atlas-based contouring is to mathematically quantify registration errors by distances between the automated and user-delineated contours through Haunsdorf or Dice measures.[36,39,43–52] As this ongoing field of research evolves to develop guidelines of quality assurance of a deformable registration solution, visual assessment through software tools such as checkerboards or lens tool is still the standard. Institutions or vendors should perform these types of validation studies when implementing an image registration algorithm. In any case, the physician should still visually review the images before using the information for radiation treatment planning.

TARGET SEGMENTATION METHODS

Besides the image registration methods, another notable challenge when integrating PET into RT treatment planning is increasing the accuracy and reproducibility of target volume delineation.[53,54] However, subjective measures have been the current standard when contouring the PET target volumes to be used with the CT target volumes. An extensive literature in the area of PET/CT target definition has been developed for lung cancer treatment.[55,56] For head and neck methods incorporating PET-CT, one pilot study,[57] which reported on patients planned for theoretical treatment that allowed PET-defined volumes to be a part of the target volume, had the limitation of not having a valid or consistent way to interpret the PET images for treatment planning. A later effort reemphasized the variability encountered when interpreting PET/CTs for RT planning.[58] Two neuroradiologists and 2 radiation oncologists independently contoured the gross tumor volume (GTV); when the CT and PET volumes were drawn separately, variation between the volumes was found to be quite significant.

One approach to reduction of this variability involves the familiar anatomic halo. The use of the halo has been reported in both non–small cell lung cancer (NSCLC) and head and neck cancers.[59,60] Measurement of the halo in terms of standardized uptake value (SUV) resulted in an observed range of 2.0 ± 0.4. However, there is still considerable interobserver variability when volumes were constructed based on manually contouring the halo edge. Despite the fact that many methods of using PET technology to delineate the GTV exist, a consensus is yet to be reached among radiation oncologists on the approach to be used. A clinician may use manual contouring methods; however, efforts have been made to reduce interobserver variability by PET volume segmentation based on a selected SUV or percent maximum threshold. In this section, a brief description of maximum intensity-based

thresholding is described for automating the PET tumor volume contouring process.

Erdi and colleagues[61] described an automatic image segmentation to determine the target volume of metastases to the lung using PET images. This protocol is referred to as the percentage maximum intensity thresholding technique, with the percentage value being used in the description. For patients with NSCLC, Erdi and colleagues[62] used 42% maximum intensity thresholding to define the tumor boundary from the FDG-PET images. This method can be implemented for manual contouring as well as automated tumor contouring on PET images. For manual contouring, the window and level for the PET images are set according to the following procedure:

1. Measure the value of the hottest pixel in the lesion shown on the PET image.
2. Set the upper window level to this maximum value and lower window level to 42% of the maximum level.

This method demonstrated the most accurate results in volume measurement for the spherical phantoms with sizes larger than 4 cm^3.[61] **Fig. 1** illustrates the 42% maximum intensity thresholding

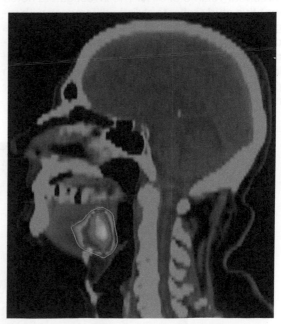

Fig. 1. Results for the percentage-of-maximum intensity thresholding method for a PET tumor lesion. The PET image is shown fused with the CT image. The window and level settings for the PET image have been adjusted using the 42% maximum intensity threshold method, which is also depicted with the green line.

method for a PET tumor lesion. By adjusting the window and level using this procedure, the clinician may manually outline the visible lesion. However, there are software systems that provide an automated method to contour the desired percentage maximum intensity threshold (or absolute intensity threshold) using software algorithms. **Fig. 2** illustrates this method by displaying multiple threshold isointensity lines drawn by a software algorithm. In this figure, small differences are observed between the 40%, 30%, and 20% maximum intensity thresholding lines. Thus, the clinician may want to have multiple target volumes drawn for deciding on the final PET tumor volume.

Simon and colleagues[63] reported on the overlap of the manually contoured GTV defined on both PET and CT for patients with head and neck cancer. Using customized autocontouring software in combination with the conformality index (CI), they measured the goodness of fit of a given PET isointensity level with the GTV defined on PET (GTV_{PET}) and on CT (GTV_{CT}). In this study, the results showed that an average of 24% maximum intensity thresholding provided the best CI between the PET and CT volumes for the GTV. In addition, a nuclear medicine physician also manually delineated the PET volumes that resulted in a higher averaged maximum intensity threshold volume of 34%. The investigators noted that this study reflects stylistic differences with regard to adjustment of the display thresholds between radiation oncologists and nuclear medicine radiologists. However, the use of automated intensity thresholding methods is helpful in providing physicians with a starting point for manually contouring a PET tumor lesion.

TREATMENT PLANNING INTEGRATION

Although integration of PET imaging was a challenge in RT planning, it has been eliminated using the Digital Imaging and Communications in Medicine (DICOM) Standard for transmitting, converting, and associating medical imaging data between medical systems.[64] This standard describes the methods of formatting and exchanging images and associated information. DICOM relies on industry standard network connections and effectively addresses the communication of digital images, such as CT, MR, PET, and RT objects. In addition, DICOM registration objects have been created to exchange the transformation between 2 registered image studies. Over the past decade, an extension to DICOM was developed for RT objects, referred to as DICOM-RT. This extension handles the technical data objects in radiation oncology, such as anatomic contours, digitally reconstructed radiograph (DRR) images, treatment planning data, and dose distribution data. Many CT simulator and treatment planning vendors have adopted DICOM-RT for ensuring a cost-effective solution for sharing technical data in a radiation oncology department. The DICOM-RT objects used for CT simulation are as follows:

- CT images: CT images taken during the CT simulation procedure consisting of transaxial CT slices
- RT structure sets: contours of anatomic structures that have been segmented by physicians, dosimetrists, and physicists. Target volumes and normal structures are represented by these objects

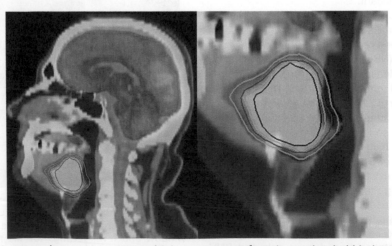

Fig. 2. Small differences observed between multiple percentage-of-maximum threshold isointensity lines drawn by a software algorithm. The 50%, 40%, 30%, and 20% lines are shown in blue, green, red, and cyan, respectively. The PET tumor is magnified on the right side.

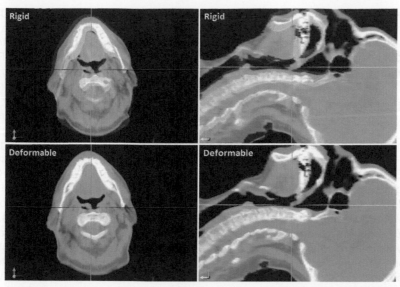

Fig. 3. Rigid and deformable image registration between the transmission CT image (moving image shown in green) with the planning CT image (fixed image shown in gray). The rigid registration results are shown in the top row, and the deformable registration results are shown in the bottom row. The image mismatch is seen in the mandible area for the sagittal image for the rigid registration compared with the deformable registration.

- RT images: DRRs that are created by the CT simulation software are stored in this data object
- RT plans: treatment plans that consist of treatment fields (RT beams) are represented by this DICOM object.

For PET tumor targeting, the use of RT structure sets is the most important for exchanging information between PET/CT workstations and treatment planning systems. Beside the RT objects, DICOM has created another information object definition (IOD) for PET images. The PET IOD

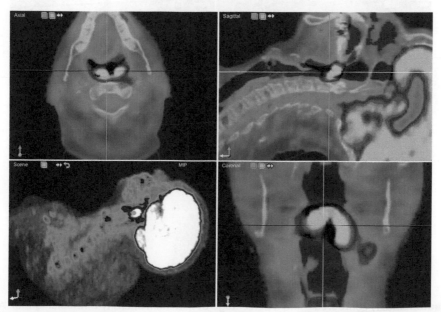

Fig. 4. Emission PET image registered and fused with the planning CT using the same coordinate system transformation.

describes the radiopharmaceuticals administered and quantitation of image data in absolute activity. In addition, the PET image IOD specifies attenuation (transmission) images used for correction and anatomic reference of emission images.

CLINICAL APPLICATION OF IMAGE REGISTRATION AND FUSION

A patient with head and neck cancer is examined in this section to present a real-world clinical example of PET-based image registration and tumor targeting using a dedicated workstation (VelocityAI, Velocity Medical Solutions, Atlanta, GA, USA). This example represents the registration of a PET/CT imaging study with a planning CT image study as described in scenario 2.

In this example, a 69-year-old man was found to have a left-sided tonsillar abnormality. The lesion involved the tonsillar fossa and the anterior pillar, with extension to involve the soft palate. Staging diagnostic CT scan did not show any suspicious cervical adenopathy or any evidence of metastatic disease. PET imaging study confirmed hypermetabolic activity at the primary site and additionally showed a questionable left-sided lymph node with maximum SUV of 3.5. The patient proceeded with chemoradiation treatment planning and delivery. CT simulation was initially performed on this patient using a head mask immobilization device along with neck pad holders. After CT simulation, the patient was sent to the nuclear medicine department for a PET/CT image study. The same immobilization devices were used for PET/CT, along with a flat tabletop. The image registration problem is to align the PET/CT imaging study to the CT simulation imaging study for target delineation and treatment planning. To perform this image registration, the user can align the transmission CT image (CT image from the dual PET/CT scanner) to the planning CT image (CT image from the CT simulator). **Fig. 3** shows both a rigid and deformable image registration between the transmission CT and planning CT images. The emission PET image can then be fused with the planning CT using the same coordinate system transformation as shown in **Fig. 4**. Thus, the PET to planning CT image registration becomes a CT-to-CT image registration problem.

Once registered, a region of interest (ROI) was created surrounding the patient's visualized gross disease on the PET scan. Within that region, a GTV contour was automatically generated using a maximum isointensity thresholding tool. For this initial volume, a threshold of 40% of the maximum SUV was selected for outlining the tumor volume. Another target volume was then generated within this GTV to delineate the most metabolically active portion of the tumor. For this volume, again automatically contoured, an SUV threshold of 10 was chosen. Finally, the lymph node was segmented using an SUV threshold of 2.5. **Fig. 5** displays the ROIs above with the PET image deformed and fused with the planning CT.

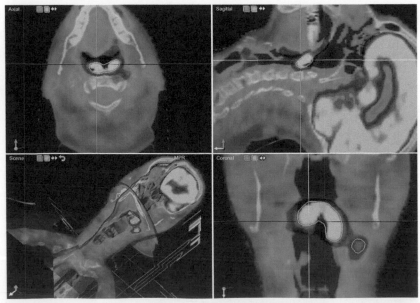

Fig. 5. ROIs automatically contoured using a percentage-of-maximum intensity thresholding tool. A GTV for the PET image was automatically generated using a 40% maximum intensity threshold value shown with a green line. The lymph node was segmented using an SUV threshold of 2.5, shown with a cyan line.

After segmentation of the PET-based structures was complete, these anatomic structures were used by the radiation treatment planning system for *intensity-modulated radiation* therapy.

SUMMARY

Functional imaging has added immensely to the oncologist's ability to assess tumors. Seamless incorporation of this information into the radiation oncologist's workflow has faced 2 challenges: (1) difficulty with manual image registration and (2) inherent subjectivity in manual segmentation of target volumes. Automated image registration methods for PET imaging have been implemented in commercial treatment planning and imaging systems for RT. Before the advent of dual-scanner PET/CT systems, multimodal image registration was a unique problem of registering transmission PET images with treatment planning CT images. With the introduction of PET/CT dual scanners, image registration using PET imaging has become a monomodal CT-based image registration problem for RT centers. The errors of image registration should be determined for each system and disease site such that these uncertainties can be incorporated into the margins used for tumor delineation. For PET-based tumor segmentation, maximum intensity thresholding allows for a more objective tumor targeting by offering a method for adjusting the window and level settings. Automated contours can be generated based on a percent-of-the-maximum threshold or by using an absolute numerical threshold. With improvements in image registration and segmentation, PET-guided RT planning will be increasingly used to assist in determining the exact tumor locations so that therapy procedures can be focused on the tumor, minimizing damage to surrounding tissue.

REFERENCES

1. Hutton B, Braun M, Thurfjell L, et al. Image registration: an essential tool for nuclear medicine. Eur J Nucl Med Mol Imaging 2002;29(4):559–77.
2. Paulino A, Thorstad W, Fox T. Role of fusion in radiotherapy treatment planning. Semin Nucl Med 2003; 33(3):238–43.
3. Butker E, Helton D, Keller J, et al. Practical implementation of CT simulation: The Emory experience. In: Purdy J, Starkschall G, editors. A Practical Guide to 3-D Planning and Conformal Radiation Therapy. Madison (WI): Advanced Medical Publishing; 1999. p. 57–88.
4. Conway J, Robinson M. CT virtual simulation. Br J Radiol 1997;70:S106.
5. Lichter A, Lawrence T. Recent advances in radiation oncology. N Engl J Med 1995;332(6):371.
6. Michalski J, Purdy J, Harms W, et al. The CT-simulation 3-D treatment planning process. Front Radiat Ther Oncol 1996;29:43.
7. Nagata Y, Nishidai T, Abe M, et al. CT simulator: a new 3-D planning and simulating system for radiotherapy: part 2. Clinical application. Int J Radiat Oncol Biol Phys 1990;18(3):505–13.
8. Nishidai T, Nagata Y, Takahashi M, et al. CT simulator: a new 3-D planning and simulating system for radiotherapy: part 1. Description of system. Int J Radiat Oncol Biol Phys 1990;18(3):499–504.
9. Phillips M, Kessler M, Chuang F, et al. Image correlation of MRI and CT in treatment planning for radiosurgery of intracranial vascular malformations. Int J Radiat Oncol Biol Phys 1991;20(4):881–9.
10. Van Dyk J, Mah K. Simulation and imaging for radiation therapy planning. In: Williams JR, Thwaites TI, editors. Radiotherapy physics in practice. 2nd edition. Oxford (UK): Oxford University Press; 2000. p. 118–49.
11. Beyer T, Townsend D, Brun T, et al. A combined PET/CT scanner for clinical oncology. J Nucl Med 2000; 41(8):1369.
12. Makhija S, Howden N, Edwards R, et al. Positron emission tomography/computed tomography imaging for the detection of recurrent ovarian and fallopian tube carcinoma: a retrospective review. Gynecol Oncol 2002;85(1):53–8.
13. Pan T, Lee T, Rietzel E, et al. 4D-CT imaging of a volume influenced by respiratory motion on multislice CT. Med Phys 2004;31:333.
14. Nehmeh S, Erdi Y, Ling C, et al. Effect of respiratory gating on quantifying PET images of lung cancer. J Nucl Med 2002;43(7):876.
15. Wagman R, Yorke E, Ford E, et al. Respiratory gating for liver tumors: use in dose escalation. Int J Radiat Oncol Biol Phys 2003;55(3):659–68.
16. Kooy H, Van Herk M, Barnes P, et al. Image fusion for stereotactic radiotherapy and radiosurgery treatment planning. Int J Radiat Oncol Biol Phys 1994; 28(5):1229–34.
17. Levin D, Hu X, Tan K, et al. The brain: integrated three-dimensional display of MR and PET images. Radiology 1989;172(3):783.
18. Pelizzari C, Chen G, Halpern H, et al. Three dimensional correlation of PET, CT and MRI images. J Nucl Med 1987;28:682–9.
19. Pelizzari C, Chen G, Spelbring D, et al. Accurate three-dimensional registration of CT, PET, and/or MR images of the brain. J Comput Assist Tomogr 1989;13(1):20.
20. Schad L, Boesecke R, Schlegel W, et al. Three dimensional image correlation of CT, MR, and PET studies in radiotherapy treatment planning of brain tumors. J Comput Assist Tomogr 1987;11(6):948.

21. Maes F, Collignon A, Vandermeulen D, et al. Multi-modality image registration by maximization of mutual information. IEEE Trans Med Imaging 2002; 16(2):187–98.

22. Wells W III, Viola P, Atsumi H, et al. Multi-modal volume registration by maximization of mutual information. Med Image Anal 1996;1(1):35–51.

23. Rosenman JG, Julian G, Miller M, et al. Image registration: an essential part of radiation therapy treatment planning. Int J Radiat Oncol Biol Phys 1998; 40(1):197–205.

24. Fox P, Perlmutter J, Raichle M. A stereotactic method of anatomical localization for positron emission tomography. J Comput Assist Tomogr 1985;9(1):141.

25. Maurer C Jr, Fitzpatrick J, Wang M, et al. Registration of head volume images using implantable fiducial markers. IEEE Trans Med Imaging 2002;16(4): 447–62.

26. Strother S, Anderson J, Xu X, et al. Quantitative comparisons of image registration techniques based on high-resolution MRI of the brain. J Comput Assist Tomogr 1994;18(6):954.

27. Bajcsy R, Kovacic S. Multiresolution elastic matching. Comput Vis Graph Image Process 1989;46(1):1–21.

28. Gee J, Reivich M, Bajcsy R. Elastically deforming 3D atlas to match anatomical brain images. J Comput Assist Tomogr 1993;17(2):225.

29. Thirion J. Image matching as a diffusion process: an analogy with Maxwell's demons. Med Image Anal 1998;2(3):243–60.

30. Thompson P, Toga A. A surface-based technique for warping three-dimensional images of the brain. IEEE Trans Med Imaging 2002;15(4):402–17.

31. Fitzpatrick J, West J, Maurer C Jr. Predicting error in rigid-body point-based registration. IEEE Trans Med Imaging 2002;17(5):694–702.

32. Grosu A, Weber W, Riedel E, et al. L-(methyl-11C) methionine positron emission tomography for target delineation in resected high-grade gliomas before radiotherapy. Int J Radiat Oncol Biol Phys 2005; 63(1):64–74.

33. Nithiananthan S, Brock KK, Daly MJ, et al. Demons deformable registration for CBCT-guided procedures in the head and neck: convergence and accuracy. Med Phys 2009;36(10):4755–64.

34. Brock KK. Results of a multi-institution deformable registration accuracy study (MIDRAS). Int J Radiat Oncol Biol Phys 2010;76(2):583–96.

35. Brock KK, Nichol AM, Menard C, et al. Accuracy and sensitivity of finite element model-based deformable registration of the prostate. Med Phys 2008;35(9):4019–25.

36. Suh JW, Wyatt CL. Deformable registration of supine and prone colons for computed tomographic colonography. J Comput Assist Tomogr 2009;33(6):902–11.

37. Miyabe Y, Narita Y, Mizowaki T, et al. New algorithm to simulate organ movement and deformation for four-dimensional dose calculation based on a three-dimensional CT and fluoroscopy of the thorax. Med Phys 2009;36(10):4328–39.

38. Nithiananthan S, Brock KK, Irish JC, et al. Deformable registration for intra-operative cone-beam CT guidance of head and neck surgery. Conf Proc IEEE Eng Med Biol Soc 2008;2008:3634–7.

39. Ostergaard Noe K, De Senneville BD, Elstrom UV, et al. Acceleration and validation of optical flow based deformable registration for image-guided radiotherapy. Acta Oncol 2008;47(7):1286–93.

40. Wu Z, Rietzel E, Boldea V, et al. Evaluation of deformable registration of patient lung 4DCT with subanatomical region segmentations. Med Phys 2008;35(2):775–81.

41. Castillo R, Castillo E, Guerra R, et al. A framework for evaluation of deformable image registration spatial accuracy using large landmark point sets. Phys Med Biol 2009;54(7):1849–70.

42. Kashani R, Hub M, Balter JM, et al. Objective assessment of deformable image registration in radiotherapy: a multi-institution study. Med Phys 2008;35(12):5944–53.

43. Makni N, Puech P, Lopes R, et al. Combining a deformable model and a probabilistic framework for an automatic 3D segmentation of prostate on MRI. Int J Comput Assist Radiol Surg 2009;4(2): 181–8.

44. Bender ET, Mehta MP, Tome WA. On the estimation of the location of the hippocampus in the context of hippocampal avoidance whole brain radiotherapy treatment planning. Technol Cancer Res Treat 2009; 8(6):425–32.

45. Hwang AB, Bacharach SL, Yom SS, et al. Can positron emission tomography (PET) or PET/computed tomography (CT) acquired in a nontreatment position be accurately registered to a head-and-neck radiotherapy planning CT? Int J Radiat Oncol Biol Phys 2009;73(2):578–84.

46. Chao M, Xie Y, Xing L. Auto-propagation of contours for adaptive prostate radiation therapy. Phys Med Biol 2008;53(17):4533–42.

47. Wijesooriya K, Weiss E, Dill V, et al. Quantifying the accuracy of automated structure segmentation in 4D CT images using a deformable image registration algorithm. Med Phys 2008;35(4):1251–60.

48. Chao M, Li T, Schreibmann E, et al. Automated contour mapping with a regional deformable model. Int J Radiat Oncol Biol Phys 2008;70(2):599–608.

49. Orban de Xivry J, Janssens G, Bosmans G, et al. Tumour delineation and cumulative dose computation in radiotherapy based on deformable registration of respiratory correlated CT images of lung cancer patients. Radiother Oncol 2007;85(2):232–8.

50. Bender ET, Tome WA. The utilization of consistency metrics for error analysis in deformable image registration. Phys Med Biol 2009;54(18):5561–77.

51. Castadot P, Lee JA, Parraga A, et al. Comparison of 12 deformable registration strategies in adaptive radiation therapy for the treatment of head and neck tumors. Radiother Oncol 2008;89(1):1–12.

52. Lawson JD, Schreibmann E, Jani AB, et al. Quantitative evaluation of a cone-beam computed tomography-planning computed tomography deformable image registration method for adaptive radiation therapy. J Appl Clin Med Phys 2007;8(4): 2432.

53. Biehl K, Kong F, Dehdashti F, et al. 18F-FDG PET definition of gross tumor volume for radiotherapy of non-small cell lung cancer: is a single standardized uptake value threshold approach appropriate? J Nucl Med 2006;47(11):1808.

54. Nestle U, Kremp S, Schaefer-Schuler A, et al. Comparison of different methods for delineation of 18F-FDG PET-positive tissue for target volume definition in radiotherapy of patients with non-small cell lung cancer. J Nucl Med 2005;46(8):1342.

55. Gondi V, Bradley K, Mehta M, et al. Impact of hybrid fluorodeoxyglucose positron-emission tomography/computed tomography on radiotherapy planning in esophageal and non-small-cell lung cancer. Int J Radiat Oncol Biol Phys 2007;67(1): 187–95.

56. van Baardwijk A, Bosmans G, Boersma L, et al. PET-CT-based auto-contouring in non-small-cell lung cancer correlates with pathology and reduces interobserver variability in the delineation of the primary tumor and involved nodal volumes. Int J Radiat Oncol Biol Phys 2007;68(3):779–86.

57. Schwartz D, Ford E, Rajendran J, et al. FDG-PET/CT imaging for preradiotherapy staging of head-and-neck squamous cell carcinoma. Int J Radiat Oncol Biol Phys 2005;61(1):129–36.

58. Riegel A, Berson A, Destian S. Variability of gross tumor volume delineation in head-and-neck cancer using CT and PET/CT fusion. Int J Radiat Oncol Biol Phys 2006;65(3):726–32.

59. Ashamalla H, Guirgius A, Bieniek E, et al. The impact of positron emission tomography/computed tomography in edge delineation of gross tumor volume for head and neck cancers. Int J Radiat Oncol Biol Phys 2007;68(2):388–95.

60. Ashamalla H, Rafla S, Parikh K, et al. The contribution of integrated PET/CT to the evolving definition of treatment volumes in radiation treatment planning in lung cancer. Int J Radiat Oncol Biol Phys 2005; 63(4):1016–23.

61. Erdi Y, Mawlawi O, Larson S, et al. Segmentation of lung lesion volume by adaptive positron emission tomography image thresholding. Cancer 1997; 80(Suppl 12):2505–9.

62. Erdi Y, Rosenzweig K, Erdi A, et al. Radiotherapy treatment planning for patients with non-small cell lung cancer using positron emission tomography (PET). Radiother Oncol 2002;62(1):51–60.

63. Simon E, Fox TH, Lee D, et al. PET lesion segmentation using automated iso-intensity contouring in head and neck cancer. Technol Cancer Res Treat 2009;8(4):249–55.

64. Law M, Liu B. DICOM-RT and its utilization in radiation therapy. Radiographics 2009;29(3):655.

Principles and Application of PET in Brain Tumors

Donald M. Cannon, MD, Tim J. Kruser, MD, Deepak Khuntia, MD*

KEYWORDS

• Positron emission tomography • Brain • Radiotracers

For tumors of the central nervous system (CNS), the ability to accurately delineate the extent of tumor has implications for diagnosis, prognosis, and treatment. Routine clinical practice relies on contrast-enhanced CT and MR imaging to characterize CNS lesions in terms of location, morphology, contrast enhancement, and edema. These characteristics establish a differential diagnosis to inform further management, including biopsy. However, these traditional imaging modalities often lack sensitivity and specificity in certain clinical scenarios. Positron emission tomography (PET), mainly with ^{18}F-fluorodeoxyglucose (FDG), has become commonplace in the work-up of many extracranial tumors. However, the relative high background of FDG-PET activity of normal brain tissue has limited the applicability of this modality in CNS tumors to date. More recently, novel PET tracers for imaging of CNS tumors have been developed. This article outlines recent advances in PET as a complementary imaging modality with implications for diagnosis, prognosis, surgical and radiation treatment planning, and post-therapy surveillance in malignancies of the CNS.

FUNDAMENTALS OF TRACER DISTRIBUTION IN CNS PET IMAGING

Interpretation of PET radiotracers in the CNS can be challenging owing to variable kinetic and pharmacodynamic properties with respect to normal tissues and pathologic processes, including those induced by some brain tumors. In general, tracer uptake can be seen as a function of transport,

integrity of the blood brain barrier, and alterations in cellular metabolism.[1] Interpretation is additionally complicated by potential tumor heterogeneity, including areas of necrosis and angiogenesis with varying metabolic demands and blood flow.[2] Although the transport mechanisms associated with radiotracer uptake are often unique to a given radiotracer and its class, several general concepts in common are useful to keep in mind.

Areas of radiotracer accumulation in corresponding regions of contrast enhancement on MR imaging may be, in large part, because of breakdown of the blood-brain barrier (BBB).[1] The BBB refers to the highly selective interface between the capillaries and the interstitial fluid of the brain. It consists of endothelial cells connected via tight junctions and not only protects against many macromolecules and toxins, but also carefully regulates ion concentrations, nutrients, and pH. As any radiotracer showing accumulation in benign or malignant tissue within the CNS must traverse the BBB, an understanding of its components and the alterations it undergoes in malignant and benign processes can inform interpretation of radiotracer images and kinetics.

Metastatic and primary tumors secrete growth factors, including vascular endothelial growth factor (VEGF), that downregulate and phosphorylate tight junction proteins occludin and ZO1, resulting in increased BBB permeability. Corticosteroids appear to reverse this process[3] and antiangiogenic agents are able to similarly decrease vascular permeability and stabilize the tumor vasculature.[4] Lesions that show contrast enhancement on MR

Department of Human Oncology and Radiation Oncology, University of Wisconsin School of Medicine and Public Health, 600 Highland Avenue, K4/B100, Madison, WI 53792, USA
* Corresponding author.
E-mail address: khuntia@humonc.wisc.edu

PET Clin 6 (2011) 131–148
doi:10.1016/j.cpet.2011.02.004
1556-8598/11/$ – see front matter © 2011 Published by Elsevier Inc.

imaging do so because of gadolinium extravasation secondary to altered permeability of the BBB. On the other hand, different radiotracers may be more or less affected by abnormalities in the integrity of the vasculature.

Radiotracers involved in PET of the CNS have different uptake characteristics relative to the integrity of the BBB. FDG, O-(2-[18F]fluoroethyl)-L-tyrosine (FET), 18F-labeled dopamine analogs, and 11C-L-Methionine (CMET) are readily transported across this barrier, and most of their increased uptake in brain tumors may be attributable to increased transport. On the other hand, 3'-deoxy-3'-18F-fluorothymidine (FLT) tends to accumulate predominantly in areas of gross breakdown of the BBB associated with contrast extravasation, although there is often some extension beyond this.[1] Radiotracers that demonstrate increased uptake in lesions with intact BBBs may have unique advantages over contrast-enhanced CT and MR imaging, especially in nonenhancing low-grade gliomas, and in the presence of ongoing corticosteroid and/or antiangiogenic therapy.

The gross morphology of a tumor may also have an impact on interpretation of PET images, regardless of the tracer used. Processes beneath the threshold of detection by a given PET scanner will likely show no signal because of spatial resolution limitations. Also, transient metabolic alterations can contribute to a spectrum of findings.

Tumors of different histologies and grades have varying rates of metabolism and proliferation. In addition, differences in vasculature can lead to variations in the amount of blood flow per unit volume of a tumor that can be associated with increased radiotracer transport. For radiotracers with activity that remains elevated in plasma over time, an increased blood volume in a highly vascular tumor may account for some of the increased uptake relative to normal brain tissue. For example, microvessel counts in oligodendroglioma are lower compared with high-grade gliomas, but because of larger blood vessels, the cross-sectional area of the vasculature is comparable to grade 4 tumors.[5] This corresponds to the fact that in CMET-PET, oligodendrogliomas show uptake comparable with[5] or even greater than glioblastoma.[6] In FLT-PET imaging of the CNS, tracer uptake seems to be attributable more to variations in transport rather than to variations in thymidine phosphorylation. Thus, factors beyond the targeted biochemical pathways need to be considered in the interpretation of images of new radiotracers in the CNS. The integrity of the BBB, tumor vascularity, and changes in transport processes all affect kinetics and characteristic uptake patterns.

FDG
Background

Owing to its availability and relatively long half-life (approximately 110 minutes), FDG has become the most widely used radiotracer in oncological PET imaging. Its use in disorders of the CNS, including brain tumors, has been extensive, but has faced limitations because of high background activity in normal brain tissue and limited sensitivity and specificity in certain situations.

The mechanisms of FDG uptake and intracellular trapping have been described extensively elsewhere. Although most FDG uptake in tumors seen with PET imaging is attributable to hypermetabolism of tumor cells, a component has been demonstrated to be the result of uptake by stromal and inflammatory cells.[7] In high-grade gliomas, there may be low FDG uptake if there is an extensive amount of necrosis.[8] Additional non–tumor-related factors may affect glucose metabolism in the brain and therefore interpretation of PET imaging. Dexamethasone use has been shown to be associated with decreased cerebral glucose metabolism,[9] as have antiepileptic agents[10] and cranial radiation therapy.[9]

Diagnosis

Evaluation of brain lesions using FDG-PET can be difficult because of the relatively high background activity of normal gray and white matter, but coregistration with MR imaging significantly improves the interpretation of FDG-PET results.[11] In addition, delayed imaging 3 to 8 hours after injection can result in greater contrast between tumor and normal brain, aiding in visual interpretation.[12] Often hypometabolism, characterized by decreased FDG uptake, provides the critical diagnostic information, as in the case of radiation necrosis, discussed further later in this article. Other nonmalignant lesions show heterogeneity in FDG uptake. Pituitary adenomas usually show increased uptake in FDG-PET,[13] whereas most low-grade meningiomas and up to half of high-grade meningiomas will show lower FDG uptake compared with normal gray matter.[14]

Among malignant lesions, low-grade gliomas are generally seen as homogeneous hypometabolic areas.[15] An important exception to this is the pilocytic astrocytoma that may or may not show increased FDG uptake compared with surrounding tissues.[8]

The use of FDG-PET in the differential diagnosis of enhancing lesions on MR imaging was demonstrated in a study of 34 patients with primary CNS lymphoma, brain metastases, or high-grade gliomas. FDG-PET and MR imaging were performed in all patients. Primary CNS lymphomas had standardized uptake values (SUVs) that were significantly higher than all other tumor types, and high-grade gliomas had SUVs significantly higher than those of brain metastases.[16]

In patients with HIV and AIDS, FDG-PET also has the potential for helping differentiate between CNS lesions that are not uncommon in this subset of patients. Malignant lesions require biopsy, whereas benign lesions often have other specific therapies that are indicated. In a series of 11 patients with AIDS and undiagnosed CNS lesions, it was shown that the intense FDG uptake of primary CNS lymphoma could easily be distinguished from the lower uptake of toxoplasmosis and syphilis gumma, although all patients in this study with toxoplasmosis were receiving treatment at the time of imaging.[17]

Radiation Necrosis

As a functional rather than structural imaging modality, FDG-PET in addition to CT or MR imaging has the potential to provide complementary diagnostic information to several clinical scenarios. In patients previously treated with radiation, distinguishing radiation necrosis and other changes from recurrent glioma on contrast-enhanced MR imaging or CT can be challenging and has implications for treatment and patient counseling.[18] One of the earliest studies of FDG-PET in brain tumors assessed its ability in this regard.[19] In this early study, 5 patients previously treated with radiation with subsequent clinical deterioration and uncertain CT findings underwent imaging with FDG-PET. All patients had diagnoses confirmed by biopsy or autopsy. The 2 patients with radiation necrosis had significant hypometabolism relative to normal brain. The 3 patients with recurrent tumor conversely showed relative hypermetabolism and had their diagnoses confirmed histopathologically.[19] Although this study was small in number, it illustrated the potential complementary diagnostic role of functional imaging modalities such as FDG-PET.

Numerous studies evaluating the role of FDG-PET in distinguishing tumor recurrence from radiation necrosis have been published subsequently. A later study with 95 patients published by the same group discussed in the preceding paragraph, noted that areas of radiation injury are relatively hypometabolic, presumably because of decreased cellularity, with changes generally confined to the white matter and with relative sparing of the gray matter.[20] It reported a 100% sensitivity and specificity for tumor recurrence versus radiation necrosis in this larger patient cohort, although details of the pathologic confirmation were lacking.[20] Studies published after 1990, however, have suggested a less robust diagnostic ability in this situation, with sensitivity for tumor recurrence in the 80% range and specificity ranging from 40% to 90%.[21] False positives for tumor recurrence could be attributed to inflammation associated with necrosis,[22] whereas false negatives can possibly be attributed to small tumor volumes or recent radiation therapy.

Prognosis and Grading

Hypermetabolism in FDG-PET is generally prognostic for poor survival in brain tumors, but its predictive value is limited, maintaining the need for histologic evaluation.[23] Nevertheless, FDG-PET has been demonstrated to have prognostic abilities in monitoring low-grade gliomas for malignant transformation and in evaluating for recurrence of high-grade gliomas. A large series of 331 patients with PET showed that, with the exception of pilocytic astrocytoma, FDG uptake as graded visually correlated with decreased survival, regardless of whether the scan was performed before or after therapeutic intervention. Patients who were low grade by initial pathology but showed high uptake on FDG-PET went on to develop increasing anaplasia and clinical deterioration, suggesting a prognostic capability of FDG-PET beyond that provided by pathology alone.[24] A similar study showed that patients with biopsy-confirmed low-grade glioma with "hot spots" on their pretreatment FDG PET imaging (defined as areas of FDG uptake greater than contralateral white matter) had a worse prognosis.[15]

In situations where imaging findings suggest radiation necrosis versus tumor recurrence, FDG-PET can provide prognostic as well as potential diagnostic information. In a group of 55 patients with malignant glioma treated with surgery and radiation and subsequently found to have enlarging, enhancing lesions on MR imaging, uptake on FDG-PET was demonstrated to be a significant predictor of mortality.[18] The prognostic as well as diagnostic capabilities of FDG-PET can be complimentary to MR, MR spectroscopy, and CT imaging.

CMET
Background

Methionine is an essential amino acid for humans because it cannot be synthesized by human cells and thus must be incorporated from the diet. Its transport into brain tissues, like other amino acids, is mediated by specific carriers expressed by endothelial cells of the BBB,[25] including large neutral amino acid transporter 1 (LAT1). Transport under normal conditions actually favors efflux from the brain extracellular fluid (ECF), thus maintaining a lower concentration within the brain ECF relative to plasma.[26] Increased amino acid transporter expression has been identified in a variety of malignancies[27] and differential patterns of transporter expression in glioma cells compared with normal astrocytes correlates with increased uptake of large neutral amino acids (LNAA).[28] A carrier-mediated transport process, driven by increased growth rate and demands for protein synthesis and other metabolic activities, is responsible for elevated ^{11}C-methionine uptake in gliomas.[29,30] However, increased uptake does not necessarily correlate with increased protein synthesis.[31] Correlations of ^{11}C-methionine uptake with increased cell density[32] and the amount of microvasculature,[5,6,32] have been reported.

Unfortunately, the routine clinical use of CMET-PET is limited because of its short half-life of approximately 20 minutes, restricting its use to centers associated with a cyclotron and nuclear chemistry facilities. To address this, other radiotracers have been developed that mimic some of the properties of CMET and will be discussed further later in this article.

Diagnostic Characteristics

The imaging of brain tumors using CMET has been extensively studied from the early days of PET imaging. An early case reported in 1983 by Bergstrom and colleagues[33] compared contrast-enhanced CT imaging of a patient with an anaplastic astrocytoma to images obtained from CMET-PET. Contrast enhancement was seen in the left caudate on CT, but CMET uptake included this same area as well as extension into the entire left thalamus. Subsequent histology demonstrated that the area showing contrast enhancement demonstrated large necrotic areas, but the area delineated only by increased CMET uptake showed no necrosis or endothelial proliferation. This early case illustrated that uptake of CMET is relatively independent from the integrity of the BBB. This characteristic has been demonstrated in multiple subsequent series and is illustrated in **Fig. 1**.

Because of amino acid transporter overactivity, uptake of CMET is selective for brain tumors.[1] Even in low-grade gliomas that may not be contrast enhancing, significant uptake is usually seen relative to normal tissue,[34] often highest in the area of infiltration.[35] In a series of 196 patients with suspected low-grade gliomas, the ratio of uptake in tumor to normal tissue was used to demonstrate a sensitivity of 67% with CMET-PET when a tumor/normal tissue ratio cutoff of 1.47 was used to distinguish gliomas from benign

lesions. This was used, for example, to correctly classify a contrast-enhancing area of ischemia as benign, and multiple non–contrast-enhancing low-grade gliomas as cancerous. The specificity for nontumoral lesions was 87%.[34]

This same series of patients also helped illustrated the relative indifference of CMET uptake to changes in BBB integrity. Patients with low-grade gliomas had no difference in uptake of radiotracer in the presence or absence of steroid therapy. Similarly, high-grade tumors included in the series showed only modest reduction of uptake in the presence of steroids.[34] In high-grade tumors with heterogeneous contrast enhancement, CMET uptake in a given region appears independent of contrast enhancement.[34,35]

The specificity of CMET is attributable to its uptake predominantly in malignant cells; there is relatively low uptake by macrophages and other cellular components.[31] Benign lesions that show gadolinium contrast enhancement on MR imaging do not necessarily show increased CMET signal on PET.[36] However, false positives do exist, as reported in brain abscesses,[37] acute disseminated encephalomyelitis (ADEM),[35] ischemic and inflammatory foci,[34] and in the periphery of hematomas. Although overall very sensitive for detecting tumor compared with benign tissues or non-malignant pathologies, false negatives also exist, for example, in a proportion of World Health Organization (WHO) grade II astrocytomas.[34,35] Also of note, unlike FDG and FLT, CMET has the potential to distinguish between a granulomatous process and malignancy.[38]

Uptake of CMET may be partially attributable to other factors besides changes in cellular metabolism. The effects of vascularity on the diagnostic interpretation of CMET-PET is illustrated by the case of oligodendrogliomas. Compared with other gliomas, oligodendrogliomas have distinct distributions of vascularity, proliferation, and ^{11}C-methionine uptake. Although lower grade, they may have equivalent ^{11}C-methionine uptake compared with high-grade gliomas.[5] Grade III oligodendrogliomas may even have ^{11}C-methionine uptake higher than that found in glioblastomas,[6] perhaps because of the higher vascularity of the former.[39]

Not all brain lesions, however, follow predictable patterns of CMET uptake. For example, pilocytic astrocytomas may show low CMET uptake relative to control regions of the brain, but in other situations the uptake is increased.[35]

Prognosis and Grading

Several studies have confirmed the association of CMET uptake with proliferation, grade, and

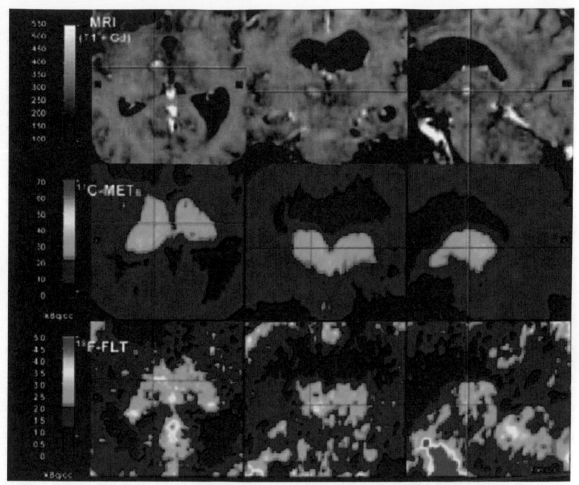

Fig. 1. Corresponding images from CMET-PET, FLT-PET, and contrast-enhanced MR imaging in a patient with recurrent grade III oligoastrocytoma showing absence of contrast enhancement in a thalamic tumor that is readily visualized with both radiotracers. More background activity, including bone marrow uptake, is seen in the FLT images. (*Reprinted from* Jacobs AH, Thomas A, Kracht LW, et al. 18F-Fluoro-L-thymidine and 11C-methylmethionine as markers of increased transport and proliferation in brain tumors. J Nucl Med 2005;46(12): 1953. **Fig. 4**; with permission.)

prognosis. In a series of patients with gliomas who underwent both FDG- and CMET-PET, only high CMET uptake was shown to be prognostic independent of age, WHO grade, and MR imaging enhancement. It was also shown to have a significant relationship with the Ki-67 index of tumors.[40] For tumors with low proliferative indices according to Ki-67, increased ^{11}C-methionine uptake is correlated with an increase in microvessel area.[5] In a study of 27 pediatric patients with untreated brain tumors, CMET accumulation as measured by SUV was not able to differentiate between low- and high-grade tumors, but it was sensitive for brain tumor detection on visual analysis.[8] This study, however, may be confounded by the fact that some low-grade tumors actually have high uptake on CMET. Other studies have

demonstrated that within a given histologic subtype significant differences in CMET uptake exist.[34,35] This correlation between grade and CMET uptake within the same histology (eg, astrocytoma) suggests the possibility of monitoring patients for malignant transformation from grade II to grade III, although this requires further clinical investigation.

Treatment Planning and Management

Delineation of the extent of a tumor of the CNS using CT and MR imaging usually relies on the volume defined by contrast enhancement. In the case of an infiltrative process such as glioblastoma, this is accompanied by the acknowledgment of the possibility of extension of microscopic disease into and possibly beyond visualized peritumoral edema. Better diagnostic tools can be helpful in guiding aggressive local therapies.

Providing additional information on tumor extent has implications for surgical resection, especially when critical brain regions are involved. In a series of 22 children with low-grade brain tumors that were ill defined on MR imaging and limited resection was deemed to be the only safe surgical option, PET imaging with CMET improved tumor delineation in 20 patients and allowed total resection in several. Upon resection, 15 of these patients showed no residual CMET activity. Subsequent biopsies of the remaining margins were negative in all 15 patients, including 3 with abnormal residual MR signal.[41] Compared with FDG-PET, CMET-PET seems to be superior for tumor delineation because of its high specificity, uptake in low-grade glial tumors, and low uptake in normal gray matter.[42] The complete resection of all areas of increased CMET uptake has been shown to have prognostic significance.[43]

Definition of tumor extent has implications for radiotherapy as well. A frequent practice for radiation therapy in malignant gliomas involves treating the postoperative T2-enhancing area of edema followed by a boost to the contrast-enhanced T1 abnormality, both with a 2-cm margin.[44] It has been shown that the T2-weighted signal on MR imaging will frequently underestimate the extent of tumor cells in high-grade gliomas.[45] As the contrast-enhancing volume MR imaging is usually contained within the T2-intense area and CMET shows uptake in gliomas independent of contrast enhancement, it may hold value as an adjunctive method of tumor volume delineation, with potential therapeutic implications.

As summarized in a recent review, CMET-PET delineates a larger tumor margin compared with FDG and/or the contrast-enhancing signal on T1-weighted MR imaging.[25] In the latter case, this may be a difference of up to 3 cm and increases with increasing tumor size, although the area of CMET uptake is usually completely enclosed in the T2-weighted MR imaging signal.[46] The area of CMET uptake beyond the area of gadolinium enhancement is likely clinically significant, as subsequent tumor recurrence in areas that had shown only CMET uptake up front has been demonstrated.[46] Thus, in addition to more accurately defining tumor volumes, CMET could detect early tumor recurrence in situations where gadolinium enhancement is not yet present.

The feasibility and rationale for using CMET-PET/MR fusion in radiation treatment planning has been demonstrated in a series of 39 patients with resected malignant gliomas, whose coregistered CMET-PET and MR imaging data were fused and used to define separate volumes for radiation planning. Volumes defined using CMET-PET were in all cases larger than those defined using contrast enhancement on MR imaging. In addition, small areas of enhancement likely because of BBB disruption from surgery often showed no increased CMET uptake and could therefore be excluded from the treatment volume. In all patients there were areas of T2 hyperintensity outside the area of CMET uptake, but there were also areas of CMET uptake that extended beyond the area of hyperintensity on T2-weighted imaging.[47] These discrepancies between the extent of CMET uptake and the T2 and contrast-enhanced T1 signal abnormalities suggests that biologic imaging modalities, including CMET-PET, can potentially inform modifications to radiation treatment volumes defined solely by contrast-enhanced MR imaging.

The clinical significance of these modifications, however, is unclear. A series of 44 patients with recurrent high-grade gliomas treated with fractionated stereotactic radiotherapy at recurrence demonstrated a significant difference in median survival for patients whose treatment volumes were defined by CMET-PET or ^{123}I-α-methyl-tyrosine single-photon emission computed tomography (SPECT) imaging compared with volumes defined by gadolinium enhancement. However, this was a nonrandomized study with only 8 patients in the arm treated according to MR imaging–defined volumes only.[48]

Not all CNS tumor types may require imaging with CMET for more accurate tumor volume definition. In patients with brain metastases undergoing planning for stereotactic radiosurgery, the differences between volumes defined by contrast enhancement on MR imaging and CMET-PET could be accounted for by a simple 2-mm expansion on the MR imaging–defined volume that would cover more than 95% of a CMET-defined tumor volume.[49]

FLT
Background

The ability to image cellular proliferation in vivo has the potential to be a valuable tool in the study, diagnosis, and treatment of tumors of the CNS. As thymidine is the only DNA nucleoside not incorporated into RNA, an analog with appropriate kinetics and stability could reasonably be developed into such a tool. The thymidine analog 3'-deoxy-3'-^{18}F-fluorothymidine is the radiolabeled version of an antiretroviral compound previously investigated in patients with HIV.[50] It was introduced as a PET radiotracer with the potential to yield clinically useful information about tumor proliferation.[51]

Cells can synthesize thymidine de novo by converting deoxyuridine monophosphate to thymidine monophosphate (TMP) using thymidylate synthase (TS). A salvage pathway exists for producing TMP by the phosphorylation of thymidine by thymidine kinase 1 (TK1), which is upregulated in the late G1 and S phase cycles of cell division under the regulation of the transcription factor E2F. Unlike TMP, phosphorylated 3'-deoxy-3'-^{18}F-fluorothymidine does not have the 3'-OH residue necessary for continued oligonucleotide synthesis and thus terminates the process of polymerization. Phosphorylation by TK1 thus results in effective intracellular trapping of FLT because of relatively lower, although not negligible, rate of dephosphorylation.[52] Uptake of FLT has been shown to reflect tumor cell proliferation in vitro[53] and calculated proliferation rates based on dynamic in vivo imaging have shown correlation with the proliferative marker Ki-67 ex vivo.[54–56]

Peak uptake of FLT usually occurs within 5 to 10 minutes of injection and remains high for more than 1 hour.[54] Circulating FLT undergoes degradation via glucuronidation in the liver, but by 90 minutes after injection, unmetabolized tracer still makes up approximately 70% of activity within the plasma.[57] Nevertheless, ignoring FLT metabolites in blood may have significant effects on calculated rates of proliferation based on compartmental modeling.[55] Rapid uptake is seen in marrow[55] and mucosa,[1] and increased activity is seen in venous blood pools such as the transverse and cavernous sinuses, the former often serving as a surrogate for arterial tracer activity in kinetic modeling.[58] Normal brain tissue usually shows little uptake, so although FLT has less absolute uptake compared with CMET, its uptake in comparison with normal tissue is higher, thus giving it higher contrast.[1]

The transport of FLT across the intact BBB is limited. Although absolute SUVs in FLT-PET for a given lesion are lower than in FDG-PET, the low uptake in normal brain tissue provides excellent contrast of enhancing tumors (**Fig. 2**). However, this selectivity of FDG uptake for areas of BBB breakdown can also cause difficulty in detecting low-grade tumors with an intact BBB. Nevertheless, there are still situations in which FLT uptake may be present in areas beyond contrast-enhancement on MR imaging (see **Fig. 1**).[1]

Compartmental modeling suggests that the increased FLT uptake in brain tumors relative to normal brain is largely because of increased transport of the radiotracer. There is still some association between increased uptake and higher FLT phosphorylation, but increased transport appears to be the more dominant factor.[58] Although FLT may be limited for imaging of non–contrast enhancing tumors such as low-grade gliomas, it does have implications for proliferation and grading discussed as follows.

Diagnosis

Uptake patterns of FLT in brain tumors vary greatly, but for most malignancies it follows the patterns of contrast enhancement on MR imaging. For high-grade gliomas, FLT-PET has a sensitivity and specificity of up to 100%, often showing uptake in lesions that are without hypermetabolism on FDG-PET.[54] On the other hand, low-grade tumors that do not show contrast enhancement usually do not show significant FLT uptake.[54] Occasionally, low-grade astrocytomas will show increased uptake of FLT, but in general they show tumor uptake approximately equivalent to normal tissue.[59,60]

It is unclear in which situations FLT-PET would be the ideal radiotracer for PET imaging of the CNS. The diagnostic capabilities of FLT-PET were compared with those of CMET-PET in a study of 41 newly diagnosed gliomas.[59] Both tracers demonstrated a sensitivity of 100% for high-grade gliomas. Low-grade tumors that did not show CMET uptake also did not show FLT uptake, but there were no such tumors that were detected by FLT alone. Of the 5 low-grade gliomas that were imaged with both CMET and PET, one was detected by CMET and showed no significant FLT uptake. The investigators concluded that combined imaging with both FLT- and CMET-PET did little to offer additional information beyond that provided by one of the radiotracers alone.

FLT-PET may play a role in distinguishing radiation necrosis from disease recurrence in patients with a history of gliomas. A study by Spence and colleagues[61] evaluated FLT-PET and FDG-PET in 15 patients with tumor recurrence and 4 with radionecrosis. Visual analysis and SUV values of both FLT and FDG images were not able to significantly differentiate tumor from necrosis, but kinetic analysis from dynamic FLT-PET found significant differences in the transport coefficient and rate of phosphorylation between the 2 groups. This interesting result should be the subject of further study.

Prognosis and Grading

Compared with FDG, the uptake in FLT-PET in brain tumors has a more significant correlation with disease progression and overall survival.[54] This is possibly because of the strong correlations

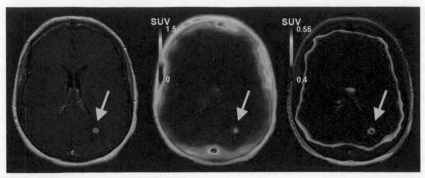

Fig. 2. FLT-PET of an isolated brain metastasis showing contrast-enhancement on MR imaging and uptake above that of the remainder of brain parenchyma but with high physiologic uptake in the bone marrow and venous sinuses. (*Courtesy of* Robert Jeraj, BS, PhD, Department of Medical Physics, University of Wisconsin, Madison, WI.)

that have been demonstrated between FLT uptake and tumor proliferation indices. This has been demonstrated to hold true even within a single brain tumor. Price and colleagues[62] imaged 14 patients with supratentorial gliomas using dynamic FLT-PET and obtained a total of 57 stereotactic biopsies. An image map of calculated uptake rate constants was correlated to the location of the subsequent stereotactic biopsies and there was a significant relationship between the uptake rate constant and the MIB-1 labeling index from tissue at the corresponding location within the tumors. However, using a pathologist-defined tumor margin, they were unable to define a cutoff value that would provide an estimate of the true tumor margin on the rate constant image map.

Uptake of FLT has been shown to be associated with grade in gliomas, but the clinical implications of this are unclear. Uptake of FLT has been shown to be significantly different between grade IV gliomas and those of lower grade, but no significant difference has been demonstrated between grade II and III gliomas.[59] Correlation between SUV or tumor/normal tissue uptake ratios and tumor grade may be more robust with FLT-PET compared with CMET-PET, but still is no substitute for pathologic analysis given the amount of overlap in the range of FLT uptake between grade II and grade III.[59]

FET
Background

As discussed previously, malignant cells overexpress amino acid transporters, and therefore radiolabeled amino acids have drawn interest in nuclear medicine. Enhanced amino acid uptake appears more specific to malignant cells, in contrast to glucose derivatives, which are taken up additionally in inflammatory cells and macrophages. FET is an ^{18}F-labeled amino acid that is taken up specifically into tumor cells by amino acid transporters.[63] The precise transport system is unclear at this time, but appears to be specific to gliomas and squamous cell carcinomas.[64] Many extracranial tumors, especially lymphomas and adenocarcinomas, have not demonstrated uptake,[65] in contrast to other radiolabeled tyrosine derivates. FET has not demonstrated clinical toxicities and is relatively metabolically stable in patients, with a plateau of radioactivity demonstrated at 20 minutes after injection, and only slight degradation in signal out to 4 hours.[66] However, the tumor-to-brain ratio may be optimal at 20 minutes, as accumulation in normal brain tissue continues for up to 60 minutes.[67] This observation of FET accumulation in normal brain tissue illustrates an important point—disruption of the BBB is not necessary for uptake of LNAA. Similar experiences with CMET suggest these tracers can be useful in low-grade gliomas (LGGs) that do not demonstrate contrast enhancement. Indeed, FET and MET have shown very similar imaging characteristics[67]; however, the short half-life of the ^{11}C label restricts ^{11}CMET use to a few PET centers with a cyclotron on-site, whereas FET can be produced in large amounts for use at distant centers, similar to FDG.

Diagnosis

Early studies examining FET-PET for diagnostic value demonstrated that FET-PET showed a significantly higher uptake in tumor tissue than in normal gray matter, white matter, or non-neoplastic lesions.[67] Subsequently, a prospective study of FET-PET and FDG-PET demonstrated promising diagnostic yield for FET-PET,[68] with FET-PET showing sensitivity of 93%, specificity of 100%, and positive and negative predictive values of 100% and 91%, respectively, in 21 patients with suspected or known brain tumors confirmed histologically. FET-PET was significantly more accurate than FDG, especially for low-grade gliomas. An additional study in suspected gliomas showed increased uptake using FET-PET in 86% of cases, and only in 35% of FDG-PET cases.[23] The largest series to date examining the diagnostic value of FET-PET evaluated 88 patients with MR imaging lesions. Neurosurgery was performed in 60 patients, and the sensitivity of FET-PET for high-grade gliomas (HGGs) was 94%, and 68% for LGG. The negative predictive value was calculated at 89%. Taken together, these data suggest a role for FET-PET in diagnosis of intracranial lesions, especially when considering LGG.

Prognosis and Grading

Prospective studies have assessed the utility of FET-PET for prognostic evaluation. In biopsy-proven LGG, FET-PET uptake has been shown to be a significant indicator of outcome.[69] Based on this observation, LGGs could be broken down into 3 subgroups, based on FET-PET and MR imaging findings (**Fig. 3**). Those with circumscribed MR imaging pattern and no FET-PET uptake rarely progressed (18%) and had no malignant transformation observed in the study period, whereas those with circumscribed MR imaging with FET-PET uptake had an intermediate prognosis (46% progression, 15% transformation). Those with diffuse LGGs on MR imaging all progressed. Similarly, FET-PET uptake in conjunction with MR imaging findings (diffuse vs circumscribed) has prognostic value in incidentally noted MR imaging lesions, and can be used to support observation rather than biopsy.[70]

However, other studies have shown significantly that whereas HGGs show greater uptake than LGGs, there is significant overlap between signal intensities observed in LGGs versus HGGs,[23,71] therefore minimizing the prognostic certainty of FET-PET uptake. This may be due to the observation that simple SUV analysis may not be the best parameter for prognosis. Signal intensity–to–background ratios may be better, as these have been demonstrated to correlate with progression-free survival in patients with resected glioblastoma undergoing chemoradiotherapy.[72] Further prospective studies examining FET-PET for prognosis and grading of intracerebral lesions are indicated.

Treatment Planning

The ability to distinguish malignant glioma tissue from adjacent normal brain tissue appears to be enhanced with FET-PET in concert with MR imaging. Pauleit and colleagues[73] examined biopsies obtained from areas of MR imaging abnormality, FET-PET uptake, or both, and demonstrated that the 2 imaging modalities more clearly delineated tumor extent when compared with MR imaging alone. Furthermore, FET-PET may be used to identify subvolumes within MR imaging abnormalities in patients with glioblastoma multiforme (GBM) who may benefit from integrated radiotherapy boosts.[68] Using a cutoff SUV of 2.5 for segmentation, FET-PET will define a tumor volume that is smaller than the typical MR imaging–defined gross tumor volume (GTV). Despite this, the FET-PET–defined tumor volume often extends outside the traditional MR imaging–defined GTV.[74]

Additionally, FET-PET can define a "biologic tumor volume" (BTV) that has been demonstrated to differ from MR imaging–defined GTVs by distances of more than 10 mm in 68% of patients, and more than 20 mm in 32% of patients.[75] Despite treating patients based on these findings, patients treated using FET-PET with MR imaging still fail centrally,[76] illustrating the need for more effective therapies in HGG. However, FET-PET targeting of therapies may allow for more effective tumor coverage and sparing of normal tissues.

Tumor Recurrence Versus Treatment Change

FET-PET has demonstrated value in addition to MR imaging in evaluating tumor recurrence after various treatment regimens.[77–79] In 53 patients with suspected recurrent disease, absence of FET-PET focal uptake has been shown to reliably predict for lack of recurrence.[78] In an additional study, FET-PET revealed a correct diagnosis in 44 of 45 patients, with a specificity of 93% (50% for MR imaging) and sensitivity of 100% (94% for MR imaging). These studies suggest the use of radiolabeled amino acid studies in addition to MR imaging to evaluate recurrence following therapy may be warranted.

FDOPA
Background

L-DOPA (L-3,4-dihydroxyphenylalanine) is a naturally occurring precursor to dopamine, a neurotransmitter intimately involved in neuromuscular coordination. The 3,4-dihydroxy-6-F-18-fluoro-L-phenylalanine ([^{18}F]-FDOPA) is an amino acid analog that has been used extensively for imaging of the dopaminergic system in movement disorders such as Parkinson's disease.[80,81] FDOPA is taken into the normal brain, across the BBB, by a neutral amino acid transporter,[82] and normally accumulates in the basal ganglia, whereas little signal is seen in the cerebral cortex or white matter.

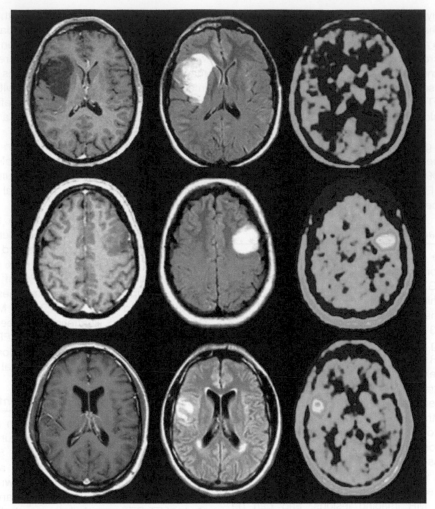

Fig. 3. FET-PET images from 3 separate patients with grade II diffuse astrocytoma representing 3 distinct prognostic groups: circumscribed tumors with no FET uptake (top row, low rate of progression), circumscribed tumors with FET uptake (middle row, intermediate rate of progression), and diffuse tumors with FET uptake (bottom row, all patients progressed). First, second, and third columns contain T1-weighted MR imaging, T2-weighted MR imaging, and FET-PET, respectively. All lesions were nonenhancing with contrast on MR imaging. (*Reprinted from* Floeth FW, Pauleit D, Sabel M, et al. Prognostic value of O-(2–18F-fluoroethyl)-L-tyrosine PET and MRI in low-grade glioma. J Nucl Med 2007;48(4):524. **Fig. 1**; with permission.)

The first realization of oncologic utility of FDOPA was demonstrated in a woman undergoing FDOPA-PET for evaluation of a movement disorder.[83] She was found to have focal uptake in the right frontal lobe, which was demonstrated to be a grade 2 oligoastrocytoma. Subsequent studies in patients with glioma demonstrate that the signal intensity peaks in tumors between 10 and 30 minutes after injection.[84] While sharing transport mechanisms with ^{11}C-L-Methionine, the longer half-life afforded by [18]F (110 vs 20 minutes) provides logistical advantages to the use of FDOPA for PET imaging, as ^{11}C-L-Methionine is therefore not available to PET centers distant to a cyclotron. FDOPA-PET is especially useful for diagnosis of

low-grade lesions and detection of recurrent disease.

Diagnosis

FDOPA crosses the BBB via a carrier-mediated transport mechanism known as the LNAA transport system.[85,86] This provides an important diagnostic advantage to FDOPA-PET, as FDOPA uptake occurs in both enhancing and nonenhancing tumors.

Following the initial case report mentioned previously,[83] a study was undertaken to examine the imaging quality afforded by FDOPA-PET in comparison with CMET-PET in patients with known supratentorial brain lesions. Both FDOPA-PET and CMET-PET demonstrated uptake in all lesions. The uptake of tumor 20 minutes after injection appeared maximal, whereas images at later time points (70 minutes) showed reduced tumor uptake and enhanced basal ganglia accumulation, suggesting that earlier imaging is optimal for tumor delineation.[87]

A larger study[84] comparing FDOPA-PET and FDG-PET in patients with glioma demonstrated superiority of FDOPA-PET over FDG-PET for visualizing high-grade and low-grade/recurrent tumors. FDOPA-PET demonstrated activity in 22 of 23 patients with tumor. Furthermore, FDOPA-PET did not show any uptake in 3 patients without active disease (in long-term remission), but 4 patients with radiation necrosis had very low but visible FDOPA-PET uptake. Therefore, by simple visual analysis, FDOPA had a sensitivity of 96%, a specificity of 43%, and an overall accuracy of 83%, corresponding to a positive predictive value (PPV) of 85% and a negative predictive value (NPV) of 75%. FDG-PET showed a sensitivity of 61%, specificity of 43%, PPV of 78%, and NPV of 25%, and an overall accuracy of 57% (95% confidence interval [CI], 39%–74%).

Additionally, the contrast for imaging of tumors was higher with FDOPA-PET than for FDG-PET. Because of the high contrast, thresholds of tumor to normal brain (T/N), tumor to striatum (T/S), and tumor to white matter (T/W) were able to be defined that enhanced the specificity of FDOPA-PET. Using these parameters in another 51 patients, the diagnostic accuracy was improved (sensitivity 98%, specificity 86%, PPV 95%, NPV 95%, accuracy 95%). There was no significant difference between uptake levels in high-grade tumors versus low-grade tumors. Contrast-enhancing tumors and nonenhancing tumors had similar uptake, supporting the notion that BBB breakdown is not a prerequisite for uptake into tumors.

A more recent study confirmed the utility of FDOPA-PET, demonstrating that the sensitivity of FDOPA-PET for gliomas was 95%, whereas that of MR imaging was 91%. Furthermore, through image fusion it was shown that FDOPA-PET signal identifies both enhancing and nonenhancing tumor equally well, and may have utility in distinguishing nonenhancing tumor from other causes of T2-weighted signal abnormalities such as edema. FDOPA labeling was comparable in both HGGs and LGGs.[88]

Radiation Necrosis

Tripathi and colleagues[89] examined FDOPA-PET in comparison with FLT-PET and FDG-PET in 10 patients with suspected recurrence of LGG on MR imaging. All patients underwent histologic confirmation with biopsy, and FDOPA-PET demonstrated uptake in all 9 confirmed recurrences, and excellent image contrast of the (^{18}F)-FDOPA images was obtained. No FDOPA-PET uptake was seen in the suspected recurrence on MR imaging that did not show recurrent tumor on biopsy, and the patient was stable on subsequent MR imaging examinations for 20 months. Furthermore, 2 additional patients with stable MR imaging findings after therapy suggestive of remission did not demonstrate FDOPA-PET uptake. FDG-PET identified only 6 of 9 recurrent tumors, and FLT-PET identified 3 of 9 recurrent tumors. The investigators concluded that FDOPA-PET is superior to both FLT and FDG for visualization of recurrent low-grade gliomas. No cases of radiation necrosis were included in this study.

Additional studies have also suggested the value of FDOPA-PET in detecting recurrent gliomas. Ledezma and colleagues[88] demonstrated FDOPA-PET uptake in 11 (100%) of 11 recurrent tumors, and also noted that in some cases, FDOPA activity preceded tumor detection on MR imaging. Chen and colleagues[84] also found statistically significant differences in uptake levels between contrast-enhancing tumors and radiation necrosis. The use of FDOPA-PET appears to have significant potential for addressing this complicated issue of recurrence versus necrosis.

FMISO
Background

^{18}F-fluoromisonidazole (FMISO) is a widely used PET agent for imaging of hypoxia. Misonidazole is a nitroimidazole, a class of electron-avid molecules that have been demonstrated to accumulate in hypoxic cells in vivo.[90] FMISO is retained within hypoxic tissue as it binds macromolecules as a result of intracellular electron reduction under hypoxic conditions. As a lipophilic compound, FMISO does not have ideal accumulation within tissues, leading to a relatively low target-to-background ratio, but demonstrates penetration into the CNS, providing an ability to image intracranial hypoxia in gliomas.[91] Although the largest body of evidence with FMISO-PET for imaging of hypoxia lies within the realm of head and neck cancer,[92] emerging evidence suggests this may be of value in prognosis and for treatment delineation in intracranial neoplasms.

Tumor Hypoxia

Hypoxia is now a well-recognized phenomenon in HGG. Early studies examining HGG with polarographic electrodes demonstrated large areas with pO$_2$ measurement values lower than 2.5 mm Hg,[93] and hypoxia has been demonstrated to correlate with biologic aggressiveness and tumor recurrence.[94] FMISO binding and retention in hypoxic cells is known to occur in this range (<3 mm Hg).[95] Indeed, FMISO-PET has demonstrated an ability to image hypoxia in malignant glioma.[91] High levels of signal intensity using FMISO PET have been demonstrated in patients with GBM, and these areas do not correlate with areas of FDG-PET avidity,[96] and may also be independent of perfusion.[97] The location of the hypoxia as demonstrated with FMISO-PET and MR imaging appears to occur at the edge of the T1 gadolinium-enhanced region, extending into the surrounding T2 abnormality (**Fig. 4**).[98] Whether these areas may correlate with areas of failure following radiotherapy will be of interest in future studies.

Prognosis and Grading

In cancers of the head and neck, hypoxia as demonstrated with FMISO-PET has been shown to independently correlate with an adverse prognosis.[99] In studies examining small numbers of patients with glioma, FMISO-PET signal uptake has been demonstrated to stratify between HGG and LGG.[100] In GBM, the proportion of tumors found to be hypoxic has been demonstrated to correlate with well-defined MR imaging parameters of biologic aggressiveness.[101] Whether FMISO-PET can reliably distinguish tumor grade in intracranial lesions has yet to be rigorously evaluated.

Additionally, other data suggest that the hypoxic volume of GBM, as well as the maximum FMISO-PET uptake, may be prognostic.[98,100,102] In multivariate analysis of survival and time to progression in patients with GBM about to undergo postoperative radiotherapy, hypoxic volume as defined by FMISO-PET uptake was found to be significant, whereas T1-gadolinium–enhancing volume, age, and Karnofsky performance score were not associated with these outcomes.[102] Further analyses in larger prospective studies are needed to confirm these findings.

Treatment Planning

Numerous efforts are under way to identify tumor areas in GBM that may benefit from more aggressive surgical resection and/or radiotherapy. In addition to having prognostic potential, FMISO-PET may have applications to help guide treatment. FMISO-PET data indicate that hypoxic regions extend beyond the T1-gadolinium–enhancing region,[97,98] and more aggressive therapy to these regions may be justified. Furthermore, the presence of hypoxia on pretherapy imaging may prompt consideration of novel modifiers of the tumor microenvironment that are under examination in CNS malignancies.[103]

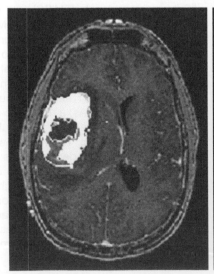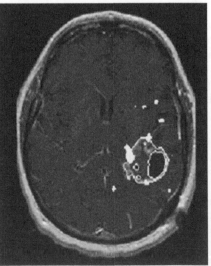

Fig. 4. Overlaid contrast-enhanced T1-weighted MR images and segmented FMISO-PET images from 2 patients with glioblastoma. FMISO uptake shown as solid white. (*Reprinted from* Swanson KR, Chakraborty G, Wang CH, et al. Complementary but distinct roles for MRI and ^{18}F-Fluoromisonidazole PET in the assessment of human glioblastomas. J Nucl Med 2009;50(1):39. **Fig. 3**; with permission.)

SPECIAL TOPICS IN PET AND MR CNS IMAGING
CNS Imaging in the Setting of Antiangiogenics

Bevacizumab is a monoclonal antibody against VEGF and has been used both alone and with chemotherapy in patients with glioblastoma.[104,105] Decreased vascular permeability is one of its known effects, reducing tumor-associated contrast enhancement on MR and CT imaging.[106] Other antiangiogenic agents have shown similar properties.[107] Aside from any clinical benefits, this stabilization of the tumor vasculature can cause diagnostic difficulties in evaluating treatment response and for recurrence of tumor. To address this, FLT-PET has been demonstrated as an imaging modality with potential prognostic abilities in patients with glioblastoma treated with bevacizumab and irinotecan.[108]

Chen and colleagues[108] obtained baseline FLT-PET and MR imaging in 19 patients with recurrent HGG who were subsequently treated with irinotecan and bevacizumab every other week until unacceptable toxicity or progression. Follow-up imaging with both MR imaging and FLT-PET was performed. Patients who demonstrated treatment response according to FLT-PET had a median survival of 10.8 months compared with nonresponders with a medial survival of only 3.4 months ($P = .003$). The association with survival was more significant with FLT-PET than with responses demonstrated by contrast-enhanced MR imaging.

Diffusion-weighted MR imaging has also been investigated in evaluating treatment response in patients treated with bevacizumab for recurrent gliomas.[109] Patients with progressive disease may have a significant decrease in apparent diffusion coefficient despite minimal change in the enhancing and nonenhancing volume of tumor, although further investigation into the reproducibility of these findings is warranted. Whether PET or MR imaging is the optimal imaging modality in this situation has yet to be determined.

Combination MR Imaging and PET Devices

Studies combining MR imaging and PET imaging in the study and treatment of CNS tumors have usually relied on the coregistration of images using software that attempts to align anatomic landmarks or external fiducial markers. However, just as fusion PET/CT was developed to address the potentials for error in positioning and temporal and spatial differences that may arise with separate scanning sessions, PET/MR imaging devices that obtain near-simultaneous PET and MR imaging have been developed to address the same concerns.

A major challenge is the fact that many of the electronics involved in the gamma ray detection required for PET are exquisitely sensitive to the magnetic field of the MR scanner. One approach is to have the scintillation detectors connected to photomultiplier tubes via a length of fiber-optic channels that allow the sensitive PET electronics to be moved outside of the fringe magnetic field.[110,111] A disadvantage with this approach is a significant loss of signal and timing information within the optic fiber channels.[112] A second approach involves solid-state photon detectors known as avalanche photodiodes that replace the need for photomultipliers and can be incorporated into an insert that fits into the bore of an MR scanner.[112,113] To date, most prototype devices developed have been for animal imaging, but recently a Siemens PET insert for simultaneous imaging within a 3.0-T MR scanner has demonstrated excellent results for diffusion-tensor imaging in the human brain.[114] The economic practicality of such a device in clinical practice outside of a research institution is debatable, but further technological refinements may lead to broader availability and affordability.

PET in the Assessment of Pseudoprogression

Pseudoprogression refers to the development of an increase in enhancement and/or tumor-associated edema on MR imaging and has been documented to occur in 20% to 30% of patients with HGGs being treated with concurrent radiotherapy and temozolomide.[115] By definition, these changes subside or stabilize over time without any additional therapy, but may progress to necrosis.[116] Distinguishing between pseudoprogression and actual tumor progression has relevance to therapeutic decisions as well as the interpretation of clinical trials. The same principles by which PET may help distinguish radiation necrosis from recurrent tumor could potentially apply to the diagnosis of pseudoprogression. In one series of 8 patients with pseudoprogression following concurrent radiation and temozolomide for glioblastoma multiforme, the 2 patients with FDG-PET scans showed hypermetabolic rather than hypometabolic lesions, suggesting that FDG-PET may not be predictive of true progression of disease.[117] On the other hand, an abstract report of 200 patients with glioma in Austria who underwent FET-PET imaging indicated that FET-PET was useful in distinguishing tumor recurrence from pseudoprogression, but did not provide details regarding sensitivity or specificity.[118] Prospective studies are needed evaluating the use of PET in determining pseudoprogression following chemoradiotherapy for the treatment of gliomas.

SUMMARY

From the introduction of PET as an imaging modality, radiotracers such as FDG and CMET have been extensively studied and in some situations may provide complementary information to traditional MR imaging sequences with regard to tumor delineation and distinguishing necrosis from tumor recurrence. Nevertheless, FDG is limited by high background activity in the remainder of the brain and CMET is essentially limited to institutions with on-site cyclotron and nuclear chemistry facilities. However, newer radiotracers continue to be developed that offer the potential of being accessible as well as providing complementary information for diagnosis and tumor delineation. This may prove to be of use when planning surgery or radiation treatments, or when trying to differentiate pseudoresponse or pseudoprogression from tumor, a problem that is becoming increasingly frequent with newer therapeutic strategies in the management of gliomas. Radiotracers such as FDOPA and FET that are taken up preferentially by tumors independent of the integrity of the BBB seem to show particular promise, but further prognostic studies evaluating their clinical utility are warranted.

REFERENCES

1. Jacobs AH, Thomas A, Kracht LW, et al. 18F-fluoro-L-thymidine and 11C-methylmethionine as markers of increased transport and proliferation in brain tumors. J Nucl Med 2005;46:1948–58.

2. Schaller B. Usefulness of positron emission tomography in diagnosis and treatment follow-up of brain tumors. Neurobiol Dis 2004;15:437–48.

3. Papadopoulos MC, Saadoun S, Binder DK, et al. Molecular mechanisms of brain tumor edema. Neuroscience 2004;129:1011–20.

4. Gerstner ER, Duda DG, di Tomaso E, et al. VEGF inhibitors in the treatment of cerebral edema in patients with brain cancer. Nat Rev Clin Oncol 2009;6:229–36.

5. Nojiri T, Nariai T, Aoyagi M, et al. Contributions of biological tumor parameters to the incorporation rate of L: -[methyl-(11)C] methionine into astrocytomas and oligodendrogliomas. J Neurooncol 2009;93:233–41.

6. Kracht LW, Friese M, Herholz K, et al. Methyl-[11C]-l-methionine uptake as measured by positron emission tomography correlates to microvessel density in patients with glioma. Eur J Nucl Med Mol Imaging 2003;30:868–73.

7. Kubota R, Yamada S, Kubota K, et al. Intratumoral distribution of fluorine-18-fluorodeoxyglucose in vivo: high accumulation in macrophages and granulation tissues studied by microautoradiography. J Nucl Med 1992;33:1972–80.

8. Utriainen M, Metsahonkala L, Salmi TT, et al. Metabolic characterization of childhood brain tumors: comparison of 18F-fluorodeoxyglucose and 11C-methionine positron emission tomography. Cancer 2002;95:1376–86.

9. Fulham MJ, Brunetti A, Aloj L, et al. Decreased cerebral glucose metabolism in patients with brain tumors: an effect of corticosteroids. J Neurosurg 1995;83:657–64.

10. Theodore WH. Antiepileptic drugs and cerebral glucose metabolism. Epilepsia 1988;29(Suppl 2): S48–55.

11. Wong TZ, Turkington TG, Hawk TC, et al. PET and brain tumor image fusion. Cancer J 2004;10:234–42.

12. Spence AM, Muzi M, Mankoff DA, et al. 18F-FDG PET of gliomas at delayed intervals: improved distinction between tumor and normal gray matter. J Nucl Med 2004;45:1653–9.

13. Ryu SI, Tafti BA, Skirboll SL. Pituitary adenomas can appear as hypermetabolic lesions in F-FDG PET imaging. J Neuroimaging 2010;20(4):393–6.

14. Lee JW, Kang KW, Park SH, et al. 18F-FDG PET in the assessment of tumor grade and prediction of tumor recurrence in intracranial meningioma. Eur J Nucl Med Mol Imaging 2009;36:1574–82.

15. De Witte O, Levivier M, Violon P, et al. Prognostic value positron emission tomography with [18F] fluoro-2-deoxy-D-glucose in the low-grade glioma. Neurosurgery 1996;39:470–6 [discussion: 476–7].

16. Kosaka N, Tsuchida T, Uematsu H, et al. 18F-FDG PET of common enhancing malignant brain tumors. AJR Am J Roentgenol 2008;190:W365–9.

17. Hoffman JM, Waskin HA, Schifter T, et al. FDG-PET in differentiating lymphoma from nonmalignant central nervous system lesions in patients with AIDS. J Nucl Med 1993;34:567–75.

18. Barker FG 2nd, Chang SM, Valk PE, et al. 18-Fluorodeoxyglucose uptake and survival of patients with suspected recurrent malignant glioma. Cancer 1997;79:115–26.

19. Patronas NJ, Di Chiro G, Brooks RA, et al. Work in progress: [18F] fluorodeoxyglucose and positron emission tomography in the evaluation of radiation necrosis of the brain. Radiology 1982;144:885–9.

20. Di Chiro G, Oldfield E, Wright DC, et al. Cerebral necrosis after radiotherapy and/or intraarterial chemotherapy for brain tumors: PET and neuropathologic studies. AJR Am J Roentgenol 1988; 150:189–97.

21. Langleben DD, Segall GM. PET in differentiation of recurrent brain tumor from radiation injury. J Nucl Med 2000;41:1861–7.

22. Fischman AJ, Thornton AF, Frosch MP, et al. FDG hypermetabolism associated with inflammatory necrotic changes following radiation of meningioma. J Nucl Med 1997;38:1027–9.

23. Pauleit D, Stoffels G, Bachofner A, et al. Comparison of (18)F-FET and (18)F-FDG PET in brain tumors. Nucl Med Biol 2009;36:779–87.

24. Padma MV, Said S, Jacobs M, et al. Prediction of pathology and survival by FDG PET in gliomas. J Neurooncol 2003;64:227–37.

25. Singhal T, Narayanan TK, Jain V, et al. 11C-L-methionine positron emission tomography in the clinical management of cerebral gliomas. Mol Imaging Biol 2008;10:1–18.

26. Knudsen GM, Pettigrew KD, Patlak CS, et al. Asymmetrical transport of amino acids across the blood-brain barrier in humans. J Cereb Blood Flow Metab 1990;10:698–706.

27. Fuchs BC, Bode BP. Amino acid transporters ASCT2 and LAT1 in cancer: partners in crime? Semin Cancer Biol 2005;15:254–66.

28. Kim DK, Kim IJ, Hwang S, et al. System L-amino acid transporters are differently expressed in rat astrocyte and C6 glioma cells. Neurosci Res 2004;50:437–46.

29. Bergstrom M, Lundqvist H, Ericson K, et al. Comparison of the accumulation kinetics of L-(methyl-11C)-methionine and D-(methyl-11C)-methionine in brain tumors studied with positron emission tomography. Acta Radiol 1987;28:225–9.

30. Ishiwata K, Kubota K, Murakami M, et al. Re-evaluation of amino acid PET studies: can the protein synthesis rates in brain and tumor tissues be measured in vivo? J Nucl Med 1993;34:1936–43.

31. Kubota R, Kubota K, Yamada S, et al. Methionine uptake by tumor tissue: a microautoradiographic comparison with FDG. J Nucl Med 1995;36:484–92.

32. Okita Y, Kinoshita M, Goto T, et al. (11)C-methionine uptake correlates with tumor cell density rather than with microvessel density in glioma: a stereotactic image-histology comparison. Neuroimage 2010;49:2977–82.

33. Bergstrom M, Collins VP, Ehrin E, et al. Discrepancies in brain tumor extent as shown by computed tomography and positron emission tomography using [68Ga]EDTA, [11C]glucose, and [11C]methionine. J Comput Assist Tomogr 1983;7:1062–6.

34. Herholz K, Holzer T, Bauer B, et al. 11C-methionine PET for differential diagnosis of low-grade gliomas. Neurology 1998;50:1316–22.

35. Galldiks N, Kracht LW, Berthold F, et al. [11C]-L-methionine positron emission tomography in the management of children and young adults with brain tumors. J Neurooncol 2010;96:231–9.

36. Chung JK, Kim YK, Kim SK, et al. Usefulness of 11C-methionine PET in the evaluation of brain lesions that are hypo- or isometabolic on 18F-FDG PET. Eur J Nucl Med Mol Imaging 2002;29:176–82.

37. Dethy S, Manto M, Kentos A, et al. PET findings in a brain abscess associated with a silent atrial septal defect. Clin Neurol Neurosurg 1995;97:349–53.

38. Zhao S, Kuge Y, Kohanawa M, et al. Usefulness of 11C-methionine for differentiating tumors from granulomas in experimental rat models: a comparison with 18F-FDG and 18F-FLT. J Nucl Med 2008;49:135–41.

39. Chan AS, Leung SY, Wong MP, et al. Expression of vascular endothelial growth factor and its receptors in the anaplastic progression of astrocytoma, oligodendroglioma, and ependymoma. Am J Surg Pathol 1998;22:816–26.

40. Kim S, Chung JK, Im SH, et al. 11C-methionine PET as a prognostic marker in patients with glioma: comparison with 18F-FDG PET. Eur J Nucl Med Mol Imaging 2005;32:52–9.

41. Pirotte B, Goldman S, Van Bogaert P, et al. Integration of [11C]methionine-positron emission tomographic and magnetic resonance imaging for image-guided surgical resection of infiltrative low-grade brain tumors in children. Neurosurgery 2005;57:128–39 [discussion: 128–39].

42. Pirotte B, Goldman S, Dewitte O, et al. Integrated positron emission tomography and magnetic resonance imaging-guided resection of brain tumors: a report of 103 consecutive procedures. J Neurosurg 2006;104:238–53.

43. Nariai T, Tanaka Y, Wakimoto H, et al. Usefulness of L-[methyl-11C] methionine-positron emission tomography as a biological monitoring tool in the treatment of glioma. J Neurosurg 2005;103:498–507.

44. Protocol for RTOG 0825: phase III double-blind placebo-controlled trial of conventional concurrent chemoradiation and adjuvant temozolomide plus bevacizumab versus conventional concurrent chemoradiation and adjuvant temozolomide in patients with newly diagnosed glioblastoma: Radiat Ther Oncol Group. 2010. Available at: http://www.rtog.org/ClinicalTrials/ProtocolTable/StudyDetails.aspx?study=0825. Accessed March 19, 2011.

45. Tovi M, Hartman M, Lilja A, et al. MR imaging in cerebral gliomas. Tissue component analysis in correlation with histopathology of whole-brain specimens. Acta Radiol 1994;35:495–505.

46. Miwa K, Shinoda J, Yano H, et al. Discrepancy between lesion distributions on methionine PET and MR images in patients with glioblastoma multiforme: insight from a PET and MR fusion image study. J Neurol Neurosurg Psychiatry 2004;75:1457–62.

47. Grosu AL, Weber WA, Riedel E, et al. L-(methyl-11C) methionine positron emission tomography

for target delineation in resected high-grade gliomas before radiotherapy. Int J Radiat Oncol Biol Phys 2005;63:64–74.

48. Grosu AL, Weber WA, Franz M, et al. Reirradiation of recurrent high-grade gliomas using amino acid PET (SPECT)/CT/MRI image fusion to determine gross tumor volume for stereotactic fractionated radiotherapy. Int J Radiat Oncol Biol Phys 2005; 63:511–9.

49. Matsuo M, Miwa K, Shinoda J, et al. Target definition by C11-methionine-PET for the radiotherapy of brain metastases. Int J Radiat Oncol Biol Phys 2009;74:714–22.

50. Flexner C, van der Horst C, Jacobson MA, et al. Relationship between plasma concentrations of 3'-deoxy-3'-fluorothymidine (alovudine) and antiretroviral activity in two concentration-controlled trials. J Infect Dis 1994;170:1394–403.

51. Shields AF, Grierson JR, Dohmen BM, et al. Imaging proliferation in vivo with [F-18]FLT and positron emission tomography. Nat Med 1998;4:1334–6.

52. Backes H, Ullrich R, Neumaier B, et al. Noninvasive quantification of (18)F-FLT human brain PET for the assessment of tumour proliferation in patients with high-grade glioma. Eur J Nucl Med Mol Imaging 2009. [Epub ahead of print].

53. Toyohara J, Waki A, Takamatsu S, et al. Basis of FLT as a cell proliferation marker: comparative uptake studies with [3H]thymidine and [3H]arabinothymidine, and cell-analysis in 22 asynchronously growing tumor cell lines. Nucl Med Biol 2002;29: 281–7.

54. Chen W, Cloughesy T, Kamdar N, et al. Imaging proliferation in brain tumors with 18F-FLT PET: comparison with 18F-FDG. J Nucl Med 2005;46: 945–52.

55. Muzi M, Vesselle H, Grierson JR, et al. Kinetic analysis of 3'-deoxy-3'-fluorothymidine PET studies: validation studies in patients with lung cancer. J Nucl Med 2005;46:274–82.

56. Ullrich R, Backes H, Li H, et al. Glioma proliferation as assessed by 3'-fluoro-3'-deoxy-L-thymidine positron emission tomography in patients with newly diagnosed high-grade glioma. Clin Cancer Res 2008;14:2049–55.

57. Kenny LM, Vigushin DM, Al-Nahhas A, et al. Quantification of cellular proliferation in tumor and normal tissues of patients with breast cancer by [18F]fluorothymidine-positron emission tomography imaging: evaluation of analytical methods. Cancer Res 2005;65:10104–12.

58. Schiepers C, Dahlbom M, Chen W, et al. Kinetics of 3'-deoxy-3'-18F-fluorothymidine during treatment monitoring of recurrent high-grade glioma. J Nucl Med 2010;51:720–7.

59. Hatakeyama T, Kawai N, Nishiyama Y, et al. 11C-methionine (MET) and 18F-fluorothymidine (FLT) PET in patients with newly diagnosed glioma. Eur J Nucl Med Mol Imaging 2008;35:2009–17.

60. Saga T, Kawashima H, Araki N, et al. Evaluation of primary brain tumors with FLT-PET: usefulness and limitations. Clin Nucl Med 2006;31:774–80.

61. Spence AM, Muzi M, Link JM, et al. NCI-sponsored trial for the evaluation of safety and preliminary efficacy of 3'-deoxy-3'-[18F]fluorothymidine (FLT) as a marker of proliferation in patients with recurrent gliomas: preliminary efficacy studies. Mol Imaging Biol 2009;11:343–55.

62. Price SJ, Fryer TD, Cleij MC, et al. Imaging regional variation of cellular proliferation in gliomas using 3'-deoxy-3'-[18F]fluorothymidine positron-emission tomography: an image-guided biopsy study. Clin Radiol 2009;64:52–63.

63. Heiss P, Mayer S, Herz M, et al. Investigation of transport mechanism and uptake kinetics of O-(2-[18F]fluoroethyl)-L-tyrosine in vitro and in vivo. J Nucl Med 1999;40:1367–73.

64. Langen KJ, Hamacher K, Weckesser M, et al. O-(2-[18F]fluoroethyl)-L-tyrosine: uptake mechanisms and clinical applications. Nucl Med Biol 2006;33:287–94.

65. Pauleit D, Stoffels G, Schaden W, et al. PET with O-(2-18F-fluoroethyl)-L-tyrosine in peripheral tumors: first clinical results. J Nucl Med 2005;46:411–6.

66. Pauleit D, Floeth F, Herzog H, et al. Whole-body distribution and dosimetry of O-(2-[18F]fluoroethyl)-L-tyrosine. Eur J Nucl Med Mol Imaging 2003; 30:519–24.

67. Weber WA, Wester HJ, Grosu AL, et al. O-(2-[18F] fluoroethyl)-L-tyrosine and L-[methyl-11C]methionine uptake in brain tumours: initial results of a comparative study. Eur J Nucl Med 2000;27: 542–9.

68. Lau EW, Drummond KJ, Ware RE, et al. Comparative PET study using F-18 FET and F-18 FDG for the evaluation of patients with suspected brain tumour. J Clin Neurosci 2010;17:43–9.

69. Floeth FW, Pauleit D, Sabel M, et al. Prognostic value of O-(2-18F-fluoroethyl)-L-tyrosine PET and MRI in low-grade glioma. J Nucl Med 2007;48: 519–27.

70. Floeth FW, Sabel M, Stoffels G, et al. Prognostic value of 18F-fluoroethyl-L-tyrosine PET and MRI in small nonspecific incidental brain lesions. J Nucl Med 2008;49:730–7.

71. Popperl G, Kreth FW, Mehrkens JH, et al. FET PET for the evaluation of untreated gliomas: correlation of FET uptake and uptake kinetics with tumour grading. Eur J Nucl Med Mol Imaging 2007;34: 1933–42.

72. Thiele F, Ehmer J, Piroth MD, et al. The quantification of dynamic FET PET imaging and correlation with the clinical outcome in patients with glioblastoma. Phys Med Biol 2009;54:5525–39.

73. Pauleit D, Floeth F, Hamacher K, et al. O-(2-[18F]fluoroethyl)-L-tyrosine PET combined with MRI improves the diagnostic assessment of cerebral gliomas. Brain 2005;128:678–87.

74. Vees H, Senthamizhchelvan S, Miralbell R, et al. Assessment of various strategies for 18F-FET PET-guided delineation of target volumes in high-grade glioma patients. Eur J Nucl Med Mol Imaging 2009;36:182–93.

75. Weber DC, Zilli T, Buchegger F, et al. [(18)F]Fluoroethyltyrosine-positron emission tomography-guided radiotherapy for high-grade glioma. Radiat Oncol 2008;3:44.

76. Weber DC, Casanova N, Zilli T, et al. Recurrence pattern after [(18)F]fluoroethyltyrosine-positron emission tomography-guided radiotherapy for high-grade glioma: a prospective study. Radiother Oncol 2009;93:586–92.

77. Mehrkens JH, Popperl G, Rachinger W, et al. The positive predictive value of O-(2-[18F]fluoroethyl)-L-tyrosine (FET) PET in the diagnosis of a glioma recurrence after multimodal treatment. J Neurooncol 2008;88:27–35.

78. Popperl G, Gotz C, Rachinger W, et al. Value of O-(2-[18F]fluoroethyl)- L-tyrosine PET for the diagnosis of recurrent glioma. Eur J Nucl Med Mol Imaging 2004;31:1464–70.

79. Rachinger W, Goetz C, Popperl G, et al. Positron emission tomography with O-(2-[18F]fluoroethyl)-l-tyrosine versus magnetic resonance imaging in the diagnosis of recurrent gliomas. Neurosurgery 2005;57:505–11 [discussion: 505–11].

80. Elsinga PH, Hatano K, Ishiwata K. PET tracers for imaging of the dopaminergic system. Curr Med Chem 2006;13:2139–53.

81. Patel NH, Vyas NS, Puri BK, et al. Positron emission tomography in schizophrenia: a new perspective. J Nucl Med 2010;51:511–20.

82. Schiepers C, Chen W, Cloughesy T, et al. 18F-FDOPA kinetics in brain tumors. J Nucl Med 2007;48:1651–61.

83. Heiss WD, Wienhard K, Wagner R, et al. F-Dopa as an amino acid tracer to detect brain tumors. J Nucl Med 1996;37:1180–2.

84. Chen W, Silverman DH, Delaloye S, et al. 18F-FDOPA PET imaging of brain tumors: comparison study with 18F-FDG PET and evaluation of diagnostic accuracy. J Nucl Med 2006;47:904–11.

85. Yee RE, Cheng DW, Huang SC, et al. Blood-brain barrier and neuronal membrane transport of 6-[18F]fluoro-L-DOPA. Biochem Pharmacol 2001;62:1409–15.

86. Stout DB, Huang SC, Melega WP, et al. Effects of large neutral amino acid concentrations on 6-[F-18]Fluoro-L-DOPA kinetics. J Cereb Blood Flow Metab 1998;18:43–51.

87. Becherer A, Karanikas G, Szabo M, et al. Brain tumour imaging with PET: a comparison between [18F]fluorodopa and [11C]methionine. Eur J Nucl Med Mol Imaging 2003;30:1561–7.

88. Ledezma CJ, Chen W, Sai V, et al. 18F-FDOPA PET/MRI fusion in patients with primary/recurrent gliomas: initial experience. Eur J Radiol 2009;71:242–8.

89. Tripathi M, Sharma R, D'Souza M, et al. Comparative evaluation of F-18 FDOPA, F-18 FDG, and F-18 FLT-PET/CT for metabolic imaging of low grade gliomas. Clin Nucl Med 2009;34:878–83.

90. Chapman JD. The detection and measurement of hypoxic cells in solid tumors. Cancer 1984;54:2441–9.

91. Valk PE, Mathis CA, Prados MD, et al. Hypoxia in human gliomas: demonstration by PET with fluorine-18-fluoromisonidazole. J Nucl Med 1992;33:2133–7.

92. Troost EG, Schinagl DA, Bussink J, et al. Innovations in radiotherapy planning of head and neck cancers: role of PET. J Nucl Med 2010;51:66–76.

93. Rampling R, Cruickshank G, Lewis AD, et al. Direct measurement of pO2 distribution and bioreductive enzymes in human malignant brain tumors. Int J Radiat Oncol Biol Phys 1994;29:427–31.

94. Evans SM, Judy KD, Dunphy I, et al. Hypoxia is important in the biology and aggression of human glial brain tumors. Clin Cancer Res 2004;10:8177–84.

95. Rasey JS, Nelson NJ, Chin L, et al. Characteristics of the binding of labeled fluoromisonidazole in cells in vitro. Radiat Res 1990;122:301–8.

96. Rajendran JG, Mankoff DA, O'Sullivan F, et al. Hypoxia and glucose metabolism in malignant tumors: evaluation by [18F]fluoromisonidazole and [18F]fluorodeoxyglucose positron emission tomography imaging. Clin Cancer Res 2004;10:2245–52.

97. Bruehlmeier M, Roelcke U, Schubiger PA, et al. Assessment of hypoxia and perfusion in human brain tumors using PET with 18F-fluoromisonidazole and 15O-H2O. J Nucl Med 2004;45:1851–9.

98. Swanson KR, Chakraborty G, Wang CH, et al. Complementary but distinct roles for MRI and 18F-fluoromisonidazole PET in the assessment of human glioblastomas. J Nucl Med 2009;50:36–44.

99. Brizel DM, Dodge RK, Clough RW, et al. Oxygenation of head and neck cancer: changes during radiotherapy and impact on treatment outcome. Radiother Oncol 1999;53:113–7.

100. Cher LM, Murone C, Lawrentschuk N, et al. Correlation of hypoxic cell fraction and angiogenesis with glucose metabolic rate in gliomas using 18F-fluoromisonidazole, 18F-FDG PET, and immunohistochemical studies. J Nucl Med 2006;47:410–8.

101. Szeto MD, Chakraborty G, Hadley J, et al. Quantitative metrics of net proliferation and invasion link biological aggressiveness assessed by MRI with hypoxia assessed by FMISO-PET in newly diagnosed glioblastomas. Cancer Res 2009;69:4502–9.

102. Spence AM, Muzi M, Swanson KR, et al. Regional hypoxia in glioblastoma multiforme quantified with [18F]fluoromisonidazole positron emission tomography before radiotherapy: correlation with time to progression and survival. Clin Cancer Res 2008; 14:2623–30.

103. Jensen RL. Brain tumor hypoxia: tumorigenesis, angiogenesis, imaging, pseudoprogression, and as a therapeutic target. J Neurooncol 2009;92: 317–35.

104. Vredenburgh JJ, Desjardins A, Herndon JE 2nd, et al. Bevacizumab plus irinotecan in recurrent glioblastoma multiforme. J Clin Oncol 2007;25:4722–9.

105. Friedman HS, Prados MD, Wen PY, et al. Bevacizumab alone and in combination with irinotecan in recurrent glioblastoma. J Clin Oncol 2009;27: 4733–40.

106. de Groot JF, Yung WK. Bevacizumab and irinotecan in the treatment of recurrent malignant gliomas. Cancer J 2008;14:279–85.

107. Batchelor TT, Sorensen AG, di Tomaso E, et al. AZD2171, a pan-VEGF receptor tyrosine kinase inhibitor, normalizes tumor vasculature and alleviates edema in glioblastoma patients. Cancer Cell 2007;11:83–95.

108. Chen W, Delaloye S, Silverman DH, et al. Predicting treatment response of malignant gliomas to bevacizumab and irinotecan by imaging proliferation with [18F] fluorothymidine positron emission tomography: a pilot study. J Clin Oncol 2007;25:4714–21.

109. Jain R, Scarpace LM, Ellika S, et al. Imaging response criteria for recurrent gliomas treated with bevacizumab: role of diffusion weighted imaging as an imaging biomarker. J Neurooncol 2010;96: 423–31.

110. Christensen NL, Hammer BE, Heil BG, et al. Positron emission tomography within a magnetic field using photomultiplier tubes and lightguides. Phys Med Biol 1995;40:691–7.

111. Shao Y, Cherry SR, Farahani K, et al. Simultaneous PET and MR imaging. Phys Med Biol 1997;42: 1965–70.

112. Catana C, Wu Y, Judenhofer MS, et al. Simultaneous acquisition of multislice PET and MR images: initial results with a MR-compatible PET scanner. J Nucl Med 2006;47:1968–76.

113. Judenhofer MS, Wehrl HF, Newport DF, et al. Simultaneous PET-MRI: a new approach for functional and morphological imaging. Nat Med 2008;14: 459–65.

114. Boss A, Kolb A, Hofmann M, et al. Diffusion tensor imaging in a human PET/MR hybrid system. Invest Radiol 2010;45:270–4.

115. Brandsma D, van den Bent MJ. Pseudoprogression and pseudoresponse in the treatment of gliomas. Curr Opin Neurol 2009;22:633–8.

116. Giglio P, Gilbert MR. Cerebral radiation necrosis. Neurologist 2003;9:180–8.

117. Clarke J, Abrey L, Karimi S, et al. Pseudoprogression (Pspr) after concurrent radiotherapy (Rt) and temozolomide (Tmz) for newly diagnosed glioblastoma multiforme (Gbm). Neuro Oncol 2008;10:893.

118. Muigg A, Nowosielski M, Schwetz J, et al. 18F-FET-PET hypermetabolic brain lesions: a correlation study to MRI and histopathologic findings. J Clin Oncol 2010;28:2042.

The Application of PET in Radiation Treatment Planning for Head and Neck Cancer

Charles Woods, MD, Jason Sohn, PhD, Min Yao, MD, PhD*

KEYWORDS

- PET • Head and neck cancer • Treatment planning

The American Cancer Society estimates that in 2009 there were more than 48,000 new cases of head and neck cancers and more than 11,000 deaths due to head and neck cancer.[1] While the majority of these cancers are squamous cell carcinoma (SCCA), head and neck cancers represent a diverse group of histologies that occur in sites that can have vastly different anatomic environments. Over the past two decades landmark studies have led to improved treatments for head and neck cancers and a focus on organ preservation.[2–4] Advances have also been made using chemoradiation postoperatively in locally advanced disease.[5,6] These studies have led to a multidisciplinary approach in the management of head and neck cancers, and radiation treatment is playing a more important role in the management of head and neck cancer.

Although improvements in survival and locoregional control have been made, the early and late side effects from head and neck radiation treatment are often significant. Advances in imaging and computing have allowed radiation oncologists to design more complex radiation treatments. Treatments have moved from 2-dimensional (2-D) plans to 3-dimensional (3-D) conformal planning, and now intensity-modulated radiation therapy (IMRT) is commonly used in the treatment

of head and neck malignancies.[7] IMRT using inverse planning produces steep dose gradients that allow for highly conformal treatment of tumors while minimizing dose to adjacent normal structures uninvolved by tumor.[8,9] In head and neck cancer treatment, the use of IMRT has led to a reduction in xerostomia and improvements in quality of life following treatment.[10–12] However, highly conformal treatments can lead to microscopic disease not being included in the high-dose radiation fields, resulting in locoregional failures. On the other hand, overdrawing the target volumes can result in high-dose radiation delivered to the critical structures that may lead to increased toxicities. Therefore, in head and neck cancer IMRT planning it is critical to accurately delineate the target volumes.

Advances in computed tomography (CT) and magnetic resonance (MR) imaging have coincided with advances in radiation treatments, and are commonly used in the design of radiation treatment plans. While these advances in anatomic imaging have improved the delineation of radiation targets, they give limited information regarding the metabolic activities of the tumor. More recently ^{18}F-fluoro-deoxy-D-glucose (FDG)-PET has been used increasingly in oncologic imaging. Malignant cells have a higher incorporation of the glucose

This study is partly supported by Health Care Research and Quality R18 CON501167 (to Jason Sohn) and Barbara Jacobs Family Fund (to Min Yao).
Department of Radiation Oncology, University Hospitals Case Medical Center, Case Western Reserve University School of Medicine, 11100 Euclid Avenue, Cleveland, OH 44106, USA
* Corresponding author.
E-mail address: min.yao@uhhospitals.org

PET Clin 6 (2011) 149–163
doi:10.1016/j.cpet.2011.02.008

analogue, FDG, relative to most nonmalignant cells. Thus this difference can be exploited to obtain metabolic or biologic information about the tumor and surrounding area. However, FDG-PET has limitations. PET has an inherent lower limit of resolution because the positron that is produced during positron decay must travel a distance away from the nucleus from where it was produced before undergoing annihilation with an electron. Also, normal tissues (brain, lymphoid tissue) and physiologic processes (muscle activity, inflammation) can lead to the accumulation of FDG by these cells, making it difficult to differentiate them from malignancy (**Fig. 1**).

Despite these limitations, FDG-PET has proved to be a useful tool in the management of head and neck cancers. Integrated PET/CT scans are able to provide both functional and anatomic imaging. Initial staging can be accomplished with a single scan that covers most of the body, thus simultaneously providing information about the primary tumor, lymph nodes, and potentially metastatic or synchronous diseases. PET is now routinely used in the staging of head and neck cancer because of its improved accuracy over CT and MR. Roh and colleagues[13] reported an improved accuracy by PET or PET/CT compared with CT/MR at detecting primary tumor in head and neck cancer patients (98%–97% vs 86%–88%). Ng and colleagues[14] reported improved sensitivity with PET over CT/MR at detecting nodal metastases in 124 oral cavity cancer patients (74.7% vs 52.6%). Sensitivity was similar between the two methods at detecting primary tumor. In a meta-analysis by Al-Ibraheem and colleagues,[15] FDG-PET or PET/CT was able to detect distant metastases or a second primary in 113 of 722 patients (16%). Patients can also present with cervical nodal metastases with an unknown primary. In another meta-analysis of 8 studies, FDG-PET or PET/CT was able to detect the primary site in 51 of 180 patients (28%) with an unknown primary who had a negative initial workup.[15]

FDG-PET can also be used to evaluate response to treatment. McCollum and colleagues[16] reported on using FDG-PET to assess response to induction chemotherapy (ICT). FDG-PET had a 100% sensitivity and 100% negative predictive value (NPV) in detecting residual disease when compared with the gold standard of endoscopic examination and biopsy under anesthesia following ICT. Yen and colleagues[17] reported that FDG-PET after ICT can be predictive of outcome in patients with nasopharyngeal carcinoma (NPC). Patients with locally advanced disease were treated with ICT and restaged by PET. Patients who were downstaged by PET were found to have a significantly improved overall survival compared with the nonresponder group (33.7 months and 44.7 months, $P = .0024$). When assessing tumor response following radiation therapy, Yao and colleagues[18] reported that FDG-PET had an NPV of 98.7% and 99% at the primary tumor site and cervical nodal sites, respectively.

PET imaging can also be a powerful tool for target delineation of tumors in treatment planning for radiotherapy. PET images have obvious advantages in target delineation when the tumor density in CT images is difficult to differentiate from that of the surrounding normal tissue such as in cancer of the base of tongue, when there is significant dental artifact, and in identifying small lymph nodes that may be missed in CT images. PET images have been increasingly incorporated into daily practice by radiation oncologists. In a random survey of radiation oncologists conducted by Simpson and colleagues,[19] 95% of respondents reported using advanced imaging for target delineation, with FDG-PET being the most commonly used (76%). The goal of this article is to explore how PET is currently being used in radiation treatment planning and to highlight areas that may benefit from further study.

IMAGE REGISTRATION

Before determining target volumes for IMRT planning, treatment planning CT and PET data must be coregistered accurately. Ideally, a dedicated PET/ treatment planning CT would be obtained at the same time, in the treatment position with the patient immobilized with a thermoplastic mask so as to minimize patient movement. However, most radiation oncology facilities do not have a dedicated PET/CT scanner, and patients often

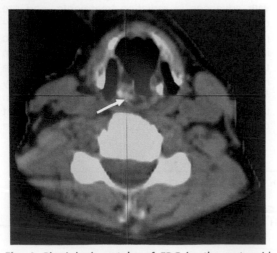

Fig. 1. Physiologic uptake of FDG by the arytenoid musculature (*arrow*).

have PET or PET/CT scans as part of their diagnostic and staging workup before meeting with the radiation oncologist. Patients are often unable to have a second PET scan for treatment planning because of insurance restrictions. PET data, therefore, is most frequently obtained with the patient in a different head/neck position, without an immobilization mask, and lying on a curved table. Therefore, accurate methods are needed for alignment of the PET with the treatment planning CT scan. Most commercial treatment planning systems offer only rigid registration, which can be performed manually or with the aid of an automated algorithm. More recently, algorithms have been developed that perform nonrigid registration and deform one set of images to align with the other. Theoretically this can lead to better registration of tumor and normal tissue volumes between the PET and CT data.

Schwartz and colleagues[20] at the University of Washington used a nonrigid algorithm developed by Mattes and colleagues[21] for use in an institutional protocol examining the use of a preradiation therapy PET and planning CT for head and neck radiation. Images for both PET and CT were acquired with the patient in a thermoplastic immobilization mask. These investigators reported that validation studies using this nonrigid algorithm showed a mean registration error in the range of 0.0 to 2.8 mm (standard deviation 2.8–5.6 mm).

Vogel and colleagues[22] studied various methods of coregistration, including automated algorithm-based methods and manual methods. These investigators reported that the most accurate method was a landmark-based system in which 4 multimodality fiducials detectable by the PET and CT scanners are placed on the treatment planning mask and manually aligned, followed by an automated algorithm that seeks to minimize the registration error. The disadvantages of such a method include the need for multiple fiducials and the relative length of time required to produce the coregistration.

Two groups have reported comparison studies of rigid and nonrigid registration for head and neck cancers. Ireland and colleagues[23] studied 5 patients who underwent a treatment planning CT scan and also two PET/CT scans: one with a thermoplastic immobilization mask on a flat table (treatment position) and another without a mask and on a curved table (diagnostic position, what one would most commonly encounter in practice). Each PET/CT was registered with the treatment planning CT using either an automated rigid or nonrigid algorithm. The accuracy of each registration method was determined by 4 independent observers who chose 5 landmarks on both

planning CT and registered CT. The distance between these 2 points was calculated and reported as a root mean square (RMS) value. It was observed that for patients who had a PET/CT obtained in the treatment position, the RMS error for nonrigid registration was significantly less than for patients who underwent rigid registration (2.77 mm vs 4.96 mm, $P = .001$). The improvement with nonrigid registration was even more evident with patients who had a PET/CT in a diagnostic position (3.20 mm vs 5.96 mm, $P<.001$). Moreover, nonrigid registration with diagnostic position images were more accurate than rigid registration with treatment position images (3.20 mm vs 4.96 mm, $P = .012$).

Hwang and colleagues[24] reported on 12 patients and compared various methods of rigid registration with nonrigid registration. In this comparison, patients had PET/CT and a treatment planning CT performed. Three of the patients had their PET/CT scan in the treatment position on a flat table in an immobilization mask. PET data were also separated from the PET/CT data for an analysis of PET:treatment planning CT registration and PET/CT:treatment planning CT registration. PET/CT data were registered to the planning CT using 1 of 3 methods: manual rigid, automated rigid algorithm, and a commercially available (MIMVista; MIM, Cleveland, OH) nonrigid algorithm. The stand-alone PET data were registered to the planning CT using an automated rigid algorithm. Tumor and normal structure contours were then delineated on the PET or PET/CT and then transferred to the planning CT. An analysis was performed by assessing the overlap of normal structures and was reported as a Dice similarity coefficient (DSC). An analysis of the distance between the centers of mass (COM) of the volumes was also reported. Hwang and colleagues reported that nonrigid registration resulted in the best registration for brain, spinal cord, and mandible compared with all of the rigid registration methods as assessed by DSC. When assessed by distance from COM the nonrigid registration was superior to automated rigid registration (1.1 mm vs 4.5 mm for the brain, $P<.001$ and 5.3 mm vs 10.6 mm for the spinal cord, $P<.001$). The investigators noted that nonrigid registration was less accurate in correctly defining the brainstem, likely due to its lack of high contrast borders and the chosen algorithm. Three patients had a PET/CT performed in the treatment position and the accuracy of registration was improved as expected. Together, these studies by Ireland and colleagues[23] and Hwang and colleagues[24] demonstrate that nonrigid algorithms result in a more accurate image registration and that PET/CT obtained in the treatment position is superior to PET/CT obtained in a diagnostic manner.

At the authors' institution, patients undergo a treatment planning CT while immobilized in a thermoplastic head/shoulder mask on an IMRT board. Patients then undergo a PET/CT scan in nuclear medicine in the same mask, in the treatment position on the IMRT board under the supervision of a radiation therapist. The authors then use their in-house software developed for rigid and deformable image registration to perform registration of the PET/CT and treatment planning CT data. Because the human body is not a rigid object, perfect matching of the 2 image sets is not possible. Therefore, the accurate matching over the entire image set or selected area should be compromised. For the rigid registration, the authors formulate Spatially Weighted Mutual Information (SWMI) image registration with Structure-Of-Interest (SOI) based weight function (SWMI-SOI), because assigning various importance weight values to geometric locations is not possible with mutual information image registration.[25] The SWMI method allows the user to assign the importance weights through the geometric space. The user can choose how much importance weight will be assigned to each SOI,

as illustrated in **Fig. 2**. The higher importance value is assigned to clinical target volumes and the organ-at-risk volumes. The highest importance value is often assigned to the volumes that are delineated using PET segmentation tools. Lower weight values are assigned to other structures so that they will not dominate the registration, thus ensuring that PET-defined volumes will get a full treatment dose in every fraction. This in-house system also allows the user to assign rigid or deformable (2-D and 3-D affine, or b-spline) image registration to each SOI.

TARGET VOLUMES

Several groups have investigated changes in target volumes with the use of FDG-PET data. Ciernik and colleagues[26] reported on target volume changes when volumes were delineated based on PET/CT versus CT alone. Thirty-nine patients were included in the study, with 12 having head and neck cancer. Patients were immobilized and imaged in an integrated PET/CT scanner. PET and CT data were coregistered in the treatment planning system. A radiation oncologist first

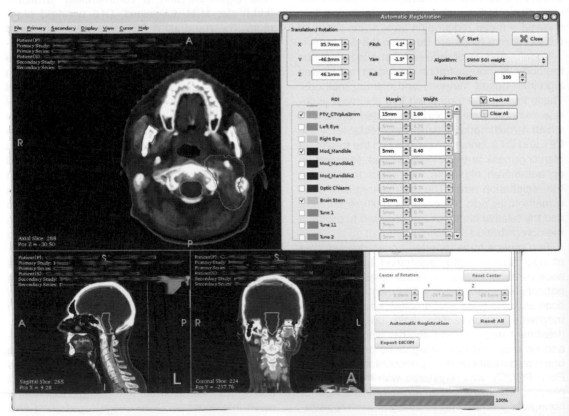

Fig. 2. Two CT images are fused by using the authors' SWMI-SOI automatic registration algorithm. Importance weight can be assigned to each structure of interest by the user.

contoured the gross tumor volume (GTV) using the CT data with the aid of any MR imaging data that were available, and then delineated the areas of suspected tumor involvement with the CT overlaid with PET using a visual method. In the group with head and neck cancer, they reported that the use of PET/CT data for target delineation resulted in a change in volume of 25% or more compared with using CT-alone data in 50% of patients. Using PET data resulted in a decrease in the target volume in one-third of patients. The mean GTV change was 32%, which resulted in a planning target volume (PTV) change of 20%. For all cancer sites, a decrease in interobserver variability was also reported. The mean volume difference between the 2 delineation methods was 26.6 mL with CT planning and 9.1 mL with PET/CT planning ($P = .02$).

Paulino and colleagues[27] also examined how target volumes change with the addition of PET data. Forty patients with head and neck cancer underwent IMRT planning. Patients underwent a contrasted treatment planning CT and PET/CT scans in the treatment position. The treatment planning CT was coregistered with the CT data from the PET/CT. GTVs using PET were delineated using a 50% standardized uptake value (SUV) intensity level relative to tumor maximum. This study found that the median CT-based GTV was 37.2 mL compared with 20.3 mL with the PET-based GTV. The PET-GTV was smaller in 75% of the cases, with the largest difference being a CT-GTV to PET-GTV ratio greater than 5.0 in 7 patients. There were 7 patients with PET-GTV larger than CT-GTV. Furthermore, in some patients the PET-GTV was not completely within the CT-GTV even though the PET-GTV was smaller than or same size as CT-GTV. When 7-field IMRT plans were designed based on the CT-GTV, it was noted that the PET-GTV was inadequately covered in 25% of the patients. The investigators suggested using the combined CT-GTV and PET-GTV for dose prescription.

Deantonio and colleagues[28] studied 22 patients and compared GTVs derived from CT alone, PET, and PET/CT. The investigators used a threshold of 40% of the tumor maximum SUV to delineate PET-GTVs. No significant difference was found in volumes obtained from PET or CT alone. However, volumes contoured from PET/CT data were significantly larger when compared with CT alone (26 mL vs 20 mL, $P<.001$). Moreover, the use of PET resulted in a TMN stage change in 22% of patients.

Several researchers[26–34] have investigated changes in GTV when PET data are incorporated into defining target volumes. The results of these studies are summarized in **Table 1**. There is a trend for decreasing GTVs when PET data alone are used for contouring. If the PET and CT data are used in conjunction, the GTV is usually larger than with CT alone. Furthermore, the changes in GTV vary widely, and likely reflect the different experiences of the investigators as well as whether or not contrast was used in the CT scan and the various methods of segmentation used to delineate the edge of the tumor.

SEGMENTATION

Due to the inherent spatial resolution limits of PET technology, tumor borders appear blurry or fuzzy. As already discussed, several investigators have compared GTVs obtained with the aid of PET with those using CT alone. There is wide variability in GTVs between these studies that, in part, stem from the segmentation method used in interpreting the PET data. In other words, variability may result from how the investigators define the edge of the PET tumor volume. A visual method in which a radiation oncologist or nuclear medicine physician manually adjusts the window level is often used by clinicians. However, this method is highly subjective. At what SUV level do we call something disease versus uninvolved tissue? Several investigators have compared different segmentation methods in an attempt to answer this question.

Schinagl and colleagues[35] compared GTVs from FDG-PET using 5 different segmentation methods with GTV delineated from contrasted CT with the aid of other available imaging modalities such as MR and physical examination. The 5 methods explored were: a visual method, SUV 2.5 isocontour, 40% and 50% threshold of maximum tumor SUV (SUVmax), and an adaptive threshold based on the signal-to-background (S/B) ratio that was specific for each case. Seventy-eight patients were included in the study. In one patient the tumor was not visualized on PET. The investigators reported that using a SUV 2.5 isocontour resulted in overly large tumor volumes, which resulted in unsatisfactory volumes in 35 patients. The GTV obtained from the visual method was similar in size to the GTV obtained by CT alone. Mean volumes were 21.5 mL and 22.7 mL, respectively. The 3 threshold-based segmentation methods all produced significantly smaller volumes that those derived from CT alone. The mean volumes for the 40% SUVmax, 50% SUVmax, and adaptive thresholds were 16.4, 10.5, and 11.2 mL, respectively. In the same study Schinagl and colleagues also examined the amount of overlap between GTVs from CT and those from FDG-PET methods. All methods

Table 1
Summary of studies reporting changes in the GTV with the addition of PET data

Authors,[Ref.] Year	No. of Patients	Segmentation Method	Contrasted CT	Comparison	Sites Studied	Stage	Results
Ciernik et al,[26] 2003	12 H&N/39	Visual	No	CT vs PET/CT	NR	IIB-IVA	GTV increased by ≥25% in 2 pts with PET/CT Decreased by ≥25% in 4 pts. PET/CT decreased interobserver variability
Guido et al,[29] 2009	38	50% of max. SUV	Yes	CT vs PET/CT	OP, NP, L, HP, PNS, SG	I-IVB	GTV decreased in 92% of cases; increased in 8% of cases; resulted in stage change in 6/38 cases
Paulino et al,[27] 2005	40	50% of max. SUV	Yes	CT vs PET	OP, NP, PNS, L, HP, OC, SG	III-IV (95%)	PET-GTV was smaller in 75% of patients, larger in 18% of patients
Scarfone et al,[30] 2004	6	50% of max. SUV	No	CT vs PET/CT	NR	NR	PET/CT-GTV larger than GTV-CT in all cases
Deantonio et al,[28] 2008	22	40% of max. SUV	No	CT vs PET/CT	OP, OC, HP, L, NP, PNS	I-IVB	PET/CT-GTV larger in 86% of cases, same size in 14%; stage changed in 22% of cases

El-Bassiouni et al,[31] 2007	25	Visual	No	CT vs PET/CT	OP, NP, PNS, HP, L, OC	I–IV	Mean CT-GTV significantly larger than PET-GTV. Larger in 72% of cases, smaller in 28% of cases
Henriques de Figueiredo et al,[32] 2009	9	Automated, source-to-background method	Yes	CT vs PET	NR	NR	Mean PET-GTV significantly smaller than GTV-CT. Mean difference 40 mL
Wang et al,[33] 2006	16 (GTV comparison)	SUV >2.5	Yes	CT vs PET/CT	NP, OP, HP, OC, L	II–IVB	CT-GTV larger in 9/27 pts; smaller in 5/28 pts; mean percent change in volume 9.24% (CT larger); changed staging in 57% of cases
Heron et al,[34] 2004	19 H&N/21	Visual	Yes	CT vs PET	NP, OP, OC, L, HP, PNS	II–IV	PET-GTV mean 42.7 mL vs CT-GTV 65 mL, P = .002; average ratio 3.1; detected unknown primary in 3 cases and metastatic disease in 3 cases

Abbreviations: H&N, head and neck; HP, hypopharynx; L, larynx; NP, nasopharynx; NR, not reported; OC, oral cavity; OP, oropharynx; PNS, paranasal sinus; pts, patients; SG, salivary gland.

resulted in significant amounts of PET-GTV volume outside of the CT-GTV. The 50% of maximum SUV threshold and the adaptive threshold based on S/B ratio resulted in the lowest volume of PET-GTV outside of the CT-GTV.

Greco and colleagues[36] also compared different segmentation methods. For 12 patients with locally advanced head and neck cancer, a reference GTV was defined on a noncontrasted CT scan with the aid of MR imaging data. Patients also underwent a PET/CT scan, and the PET data were registered with the treatment CT scan. PET-GTVs were then defined using the following methods: visual inspection, an absolute SUV threshold of 2.5, 50% of maximum SUV, and an iterative segmentation algorithm. Mean tumor volumes obtained from each method were 75.5, 57.6, 60, 16.8, and 26.1 mL for CT, visual inspection, absolute SUV 2.5, 50% of maximum threshold, and iterative algorithm, respectively. The visual and absolute threshold SUV 2.5 did not result in statistically significantly different volumes when compared with the GTV defined by CT. The volumes derived from 50% of maximal SUV threshold or the iterative algorithm resulted in smaller volumes when compared with the CT-GTV in all cases.

At the authors' institution, their in-house software uses an adaptive threshold based on the S/B ratio. Daisne and colleagues[37] considered the relationship between S/B ratio and isoactivity level for volume segmentation. Their method provides better accuracy for small and/or poorly contrasted lesions. The authors' software calculates the S/B ratio and allows the user to define interactively using a mouse by drawing a line from the highest density to the lowest signal area, as shown in **Fig. 3**. Initially, the software automatically decides the threshold by considering S/B ratio estimation. Then contours for the tumor volumes are generated by a region growing algorithm.[38] The software has an option for the user to change the threshold.

PATHOLOGY CORRELATION

To better understand the optimal SUV values for GTV delineation using PET data, some investigators have correlated GTVs with pathologic specimens. Comparison of PET-GTVs with CT-GTVs has limited value unless it is in the context of pathology and true disease. When interpreting these reports, it is important to be aware of how the tissue was processed for pathology. Fixation with formalin-based methods can lead to significant tissue shrinkage, which has been shown to cause stage migration in non–small cell lung cancer patients.[39]

Burri and colleagues[40] correlated GTVs derived from different segmentation methods using SUV from PET scans with pathologic specimens, studying 28 tumors in 18 patients with head and neck cancers. Surgical specimens were processed in a formalin-based manner. A nuclear medicine physician defined a GTV based on CT and PET using predefined SUV cutoff models: default software window (SUVdef), source-to-background method in which the limits of the window were decreased by 1 standard deviation (SUV-1SD), a threshold of SUV 2.5 or greater (SUV2.5), or a threshold of 40% (SUV40) of maximum SUV. The investigators reported that PET was superior to CT for detecting primary tumors with a sensitivity of 94% and 82%, respectively, and superior for staging of the neck with a sensitivity of 90% and 67%, respectively. Specificity for staging of the neck was 78% for both PET and CT. Pathology data were available for 12 tumors. The SUV2.5 and SUV40 methods of defining GTV were the most likely to overestimate tumor volume but, importantly, were also the least likely to underestimate tumor volume. SUVdef and SUV-1SD methods tended to overestimate less but also led to a greater underestimation of tumor volumes that clinically could lead to treatment failure. Burri and colleagues concluded that the threshold cutoff of 40% of maximum SUV was the best delineation method. This study showed excellent sensitivity of PET/CT in the ability to detect tumor and suggests that using an SUV threshold of 40% of maximal SUV may be ideal for creating GTVs. However, tumor volumes may have been significantly smaller, due to formalin processing that introduces error to the correlation.

Daisne and colleagues[41] reported on the pathological correlation of CT, PET, and MR imaging in patients with SCCA of the oropharynx, hypopharynx, or larynx. Surgical specimens were processed in a gelatin solution to minimize tissue shrinkage. Patients underwent CT, MR imaging, and PET scans, and one investigator delineated GTVs based on MR and CT. PET-GTV was automatically delineated using an S/B ratio algorithm. Of the 29 patients included in the study, 9 patients had a surgical specimen for comparison. For oropharyngeal tumors, the GTVs contoured using CT or MR imaging were significantly larger (73% and 64%, respectively) than GTVs contoured on PET. No significant differences were noted between MR and CT contours. No contours were noted to have total overlap. Similar results were noted for hypopharyngeal and laryngeal tumors. When GTVs were compared with surgical specimens from laryngectomies of 9 patients, the mean GTVs from CT (20.8 mL), PET (16.3 mL),

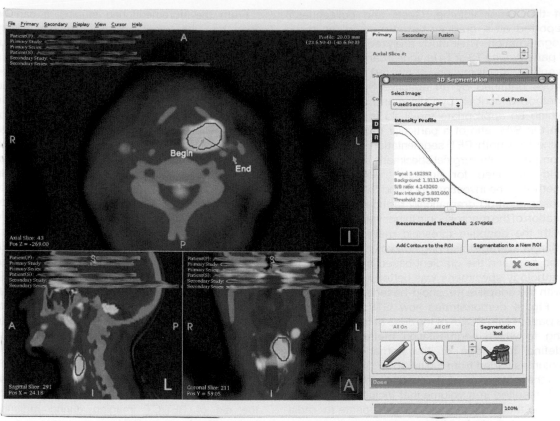

Fig. 3. PET:CT fused image. Once a user draws a line from the highest density to the lowest signal area, the software calculates the signal-to-background (S/B) ratio and determines the appropriate threshold. The user can interactively modify the parameters in the 3-D segmentation pop-up window if necessary.

and MR imaging (23.8 mL) were significantly larger than the surgical specimen (12.6 mL). All modalities resulted in overestimation of tumor volume; PET resulted in the lowest, with 46% overestimation. It was noted that all modalities underestimated superficial tumors.

Seitz and colleagues[42] used pathology correlation to compare GTVs delineated from PET/CT and MR imaging in a study of 66 patients with oral or oropharyngeal cancer, 25 of whom had recurrent disease. Pathology specimens were prepared in a gelatin solution to minimize shrinkage. For PET, GTVs of the primary tumor were delineated automatically using a SUV threshold of 3.5. MR imaging GTVs were delineated by 2 senior radiologists using a set of predetermined criteria. There were no statistically significant differences between the two modalities at detecting disease. The specificity of correctly detecting the primary disease with MR imaging and PET/CT was 100% and 96.7%, respectively. Both modalities detected all primary tumors in patients with recurrent disease. For detecting nodal disease MR imaging and PET/CT had a

sensitivity/specificity of 88.3%/74% and 83.8%/74%, respectively. The mean GTVs from pathology, MR imaging, and PET/CT were 16.6, 17.6, and 18.8 mL, respectively. These differences between the 3 methods were statistically significant. MR imaging and PET/CT overestimated the T stage in 18% and 22% of cases, respectively. More clinically relevant to tumor control, both modalities underestimated T stage in 8% and 12% of cases, respectively. Seitz and colleagues found no difference in the detection of the primary tumor by MR or PET/CT, and overestimation and underestimation of T stage were similar between the two modalities. The results of this study differ from those of Daisne and colleagues,[41] who showed that PET demonstrated a smaller GTV than MR imaging. However, the investigators studied different disease sites and used different segmentation methods to delineate PET volumes.

Absolute threshold and percentages of maximum SUV are more straightforward to apply to treatment planning, but new algorithms taking into account S/B ratio and how rapidly the signal falls off are being developed to delineate the edge of the tumor volume. Geets and colleagues[43] reported on a gradient-based method for image segmentation. Their study analyzed this method in 7 patients with T3 or T4 laryngeal cancer who underwent laryngectomy, and compared the results with those obtained by an adaptive threshold–based method described by Daisne and colleagues[37] in which an appropriate threshold is chosen based on the S/B ratio of a particular case.[43] GTVs obtained by both PET segmentation methods were compared with surgical specimens that were frozen and sectioned for analysis (nonformalin-based method). The investigators found that the gradient-based method dramatically reduced the overestimation of the macroscopic tumor volume compared with the adaptive threshold method, but led to a larger average false-negative volume. The correlation between the gradient-based method and the pathology specimens was better when compared with the adaptive threshold–based method.

Fig. 4 demonstrates how GTVs can differ in a patient with SCCA of the base of tongue, according to which segmentation method is used to define the edge of the primary tumor. GTV volumes varied from 5.0 mL to 77.3 mL depending on the method used. An absolute threshold of SUV 2.5 resulted in a volume that included uninvolved tissue that would be not be appropriate for radiation treatment planning.

From the aforementioned studies, it can be seen that the tumor volume can vary widely according to the segmentation methods used. However, the usefulness of this is limited unless it is in the context of pathology, which should be our gold standard. Burri and colleagues[40] showed that a threshold of 40% maximal SUV results in a good balance of not underestimating the tumor volume while improving on the visual and absolute SUV threshold methods. Newer gradient and adaptive threshold methods are promising, but need to be validated by surgical specimens in other subsites.

TREATMENT OUTCOMES

The use of FDG-PET imaging results in differing target volumes, but it is important to understand the influence of PET imaging on patient outcomes. Does the use of PET imaging for radiation treatment planning improve patient outcomes, including tumor control and quality of life? Unfortunately, there are no randomized trials comparing radiation treatment planning with or without the aid of FDG-PET imaging. Vernon and colleagues[44] reported on the outcomes of 42 patients treated with definitive radiation or chemoradiation with the aid of PET/CT imaging during radiation treatment planning. GTVs were contoured by

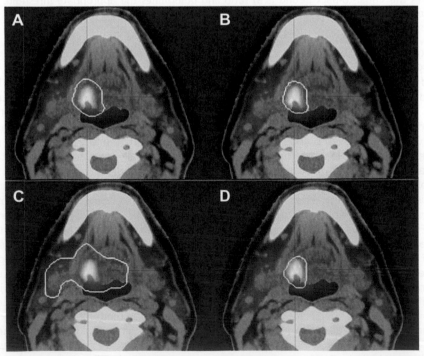

Fig. 4. SCCA of the base of tongue. Automated segmentation and creation of the primary tumor GTV based on SUV values: (A) 40% of max. SUV (12.9 mL); (B) 50% of max. SUV (7.1 mL); (C) absolute threshold of SUV 2.5 (77.3 mL); (D) gradient-based algorithm (5.0 mL). Performed using MIMVista software.

a radiation oncologist and head-and-neck radiologist using an SUV threshold of 2.5. Eighty-six percent of patients had stage III or IV disease and 83% of patients were treated with an IMRT technique, with the remainder treated with a 3-D conformal technique. With a median follow-up of 32 months the 2-year overall survival and disease-free survival were 82.8% and 71%, respectively. Six patients experienced local failures with a 2-year locoregional control rate of 85.7%. All failures were among stage III and IV patients. No correlation was reported between local failure and maximum SUV of the primary tumor or nodes, but the analysis was limited by the small number of failures. Although only 86% of patients in this study were treated with IMRT, results appear comparable with recent IMRT outcomes data. Yao and colleagues[45] reported a similar 2-year overall survival of 85% in patients treated with definitive or postoperative IMRT. Chao and colleagues[46] reported a 2-year actuarial rate of locoregional control of 85% in patients treated with definitive or postoperative IMRT. These data are similar to those for the outcomes of patients treated using PET-aided radiation treatment planning reported by Vernon and colleagues.[44] Further clinical trials with longer follow-up and incorporation of quality-of-life measurements are needed to determine the role of using FDG PET in radiation treatment planning in head and neck cancer patients.

NEW DIRECTIONS
Subvolume Delineation and Dose Escalation

Traditionally the GTV, including the primary tumor and nodal volumes, are contoured in the treatment planning CT with or without the aid of additional imaging modalities. An attempt is then made to prescribe a homogeneous dose to the PTVs. Most locoregional failures of head and neck cancer treated with IMRT occur in the high-dose regions,[45–47] suggesting that the radiation dose delivered may not be high enough and that dose escalation is needed to better control the tumor. However, dose escalation to a large treatment volume may not always be feasible and could cause significant toxicities. Tumors are not homogeneous structures, and there are areas inside the tumor that may harbor more aggressive cancer cells. With the dose-painting capability of IMRT, a higher radiation dose can be delivered to tumor subvolumes that may be more radioresistant. FDG-avid regions in the tumor have been shown to be correlated with hypoxia that is associated with tumor radioresistance.[48,49] Higher pretreatment SUVs are associated with worse

treatment outcomes, including a worse disease-free survival and a decrease in local control.[50–52] Therefore, some groups have investigated the use of PET imaging to define a subvolume for dose escalation.

Schwartz and colleagues[20] studied theoretical IMRT models using PET-derived volumes as compared with CT-derived volumes in 20 head and neck cancer patients. Patients underwent a contrasted CT scan and a PET scan while immobilized in the treatment position. CT and PET images were coregistered using a nonrigid algorithm. GTV-CT was derived from the CT data by radiologists who were blinded to the PET data, and GTV-PET was derived from the PET/CT data by nuclear medicine physicians using a visual method. Theoretical IMRT plans were constructed to deliver 66 Gy in 30 fractions to the PTV. These investigators reported a significantly decreased mean contralateral parotid gland dose and mean larynx dose with PET/CT-directed IMRT as compared with CT-directed IMRT. In 5 patients, a theoretical dose escalation plan was generated to deliver a boost to GTV-PET in a stepwise fashion with incremental 2.2-Gy fractions. It was found that a mean dose of 74.9 Gy (range, 71.53–80.98 Gy) could be delivered without overdosing the adjacent critical structures.

Madani and colleagues[53] conducted a phase 1 study of dose escalation to FDG-avid subvolumes. Patients underwent contrasted CT and PET scans of the head and neck immobilized in a mask. PET images were manually coregistered with CT data. CT-GTVs were delineated manually by investigators and PET-GTVs were delineated via an automated algorithm using a source to background method.[37] Dose escalation to the FDG-avid subvolumes was performed using an upfront, simultaneously integrated boost with IMRT. The IMRT was delivered in 2 phases. The first phase was delivered to a focal region defined by PET within the GTV with dose escalation at 2 levels: Group I (25 Gy in 10 fractions) and Group II (30 Gy in 10 fractions). Standard IMRT consisting of 22 fractions of 2.16 Gy was then given following the upfront boost with total doses delivered to PET subvolumes being 72.5 Gy and 77.5 Gy, respectively. In Group II the investigators limited the volume that could receive the 3.0-Gy daily boost to 10 mL. If that volume was exceeded, the remaining volume received a 2.5-Gy daily boost. Macroscopic tumor on CT and enlarged lymph nodes were treated with 69 Gy and elective nodal areas were treated with 56 Gy. Toxicity was scored using NCI Common Toxicity Criteria, version 2.0. A total of 41 patients were enrolled, 23 patients in Group I and 18 patients in

Group II. Nine of 23 patients in Group I and 14 of 18 patients in Group II also received concurrent cisplatin-based chemotherapy. Thirty-nine patients completed treatment, only 2 of whom required treatment breaks. Of the two patients requiring breaks, one was due to Grade 4 skin toxicity (5 day break) and the other was due to Grade 3 dysphagia requiring percutaneous endoscopic gastrostomy tube placement (10-day break). Skin toxicity of Grade 2 or higher was the most common acute toxicity. Twenty-six percent of patients in Group I and 56% of patients in Group II required hospitalization at some point during treatment. One patient with locally advanced oropharyngeal cancer receiving concurrent chemotherapy died during treatment at 53 Gy because of sepsis, which halted further enrollment as per protocol. No patients experienced any late Grade 4 toxicities. Fibrosis and dysphagia were the most common late toxicities, with dysphagia Grades 1 to 3 occurring in 50% and 90% of patients in Groups I and II, respectively. A complete tumor response was seen in 85.7% of Group I patients and 81.2% of Group II patients. The actuarial overall survival at 1 year was 82% in Group I and 54% in Group II ($P = .06$). The patients in Group II tended to have larger GTVs, and had more laryngeal and pharyngeal tumors. Locoregional control at 1 year was 85% and 87%, respectively. Seven patients had a local recurrence. More than half (4/7) local recurrences occurred inside the PET-GTV defined area that received the dose escalation, suggesting that FDG-PET could be used to detect relapse-prone regions. This study highlights the feasibility of dose escalation to a PET-defined subvolume. The investigators are planning a randomized phase 2 trial comparing the dose prescription at dose level II with standard IMRT.

Use of Other Tracers

FDG is the most frequently used radiopharmaceutical for PET imaging. It is widely available and has a clinically practical half-life of 110 minutes. However, FDG has limitations including normal physiologic uptake in brain, kidney, active muscle, lymphoid tissues, brown fat, and inflamed tissues. In the head and neck region, lymphoid tissues in the tonsils and base of tongue often have increased FDG uptake, which may lead to an overestimation of the tumor volume based on FDG uptake. An ideal replacement would be more specific for malignancy than FDG while being widely available and having an acceptable half-life.

Methionine has been shown to reflect increased amino acid transport and protein synthesis in malignant tissue. Geets and colleagues[54] compared GTVs derived from ^{11}C-methionine–PET (MET-PET) with those derived from CT and FDG-PET. GTVs from PET images were delineated using an adaptive threshold method that took into account the S/B ratio. With 23 patients, they reported no significant difference between the volumes delineated from CT alone versus MET-PET in laryngeal and oropharyngeal tumors. However, as noted in other studies, FDG-PET volumes were significantly smaller when compared with CT alone. The investigators suggested that the larger MET-PET volumes were likely attributable to high physiologic uptake in the submandibular glands, mucosa, and bone marrow.

Several investigators have performed feasibility studies using hypoxic tracers to define subvolumes for dose escalation to the hypoxic component of the tumor. Because hypoxia is related to radioresistance and the hypoxic area in the tumor may contain more aggressive and radioresistant cancer cells, a higher dose to the hypoxic volume might lead to improved local control. Several hypoxia radiotracers have been developed. Theoretically these tracers are bioreductive molecules that accept an election in the reductive/hypoxic environment of a tumor, with the resultant reduced molecule being unable to leave the malignant cell.

Chao and colleagues[55] studied the hypoxia tracer [[60]Cu]Cu(II)-diacetylbis(N4-methylthiosemicarbazone) (Cu-ATSM). A theoretical IMRT dose escalation plan was constructed using a hypoxic subvolume defined by Cu-ATSM–PET in a patient with a tonsil/base of tongue cancer. A threshold of twice the background uptake in neck muscle was used to define the hypoxic volume. The theoretical plan was able to successfully deliver 80 Gy in 35 fractions to the subvolume while maintaining normal structure constraints.

Grosu and colleagues[56] studied the hypoxia tracer ^{18}F-fluoroazomycin arabinoside (FAZA) in 18 head and neck cancer patients. GTVs delineated on CT were compared with subvolumes corresponding to FAZA-PET imaging using an SUV larger than 50% of the mean SUV in neck muscle as the delineation method. Theoretical IMRT plans were constructed to provide a boost to total dose of 80.5 Gy to the hypoxic subvolumes. The investigators were able to delineate a hypoxic subvolume for the primary tumor in 15 of 18 patients. The FAZA-GTV for the primary tumor failed to correlate significantly with the CT-GTV, and represented only a median of 10.8% of the CT-GTV (range 0.7%–52.0%). For the lymph nodes, hypoxic subvolumes were able to be delineated in only 10 of 16 patients. In contrast to the primary tumors, the nodal hypoxic subvolumes correlated significantly with the nodal CT-GTVs. In 22% of patients, the hypoxic subvolumes were not contiguous, as would be expected; this could have led to the lack of correlation between GTV-FAZA and GTV-CT in the primary tumor. Grosu and colleagues also showed that the theoretical IMRT plan giving 80.5 Gy to the hypoxic subvolume did not increase radiation dose to the critical structures.

Lee and colleagues[57] studied the feasibility of dose escalation to subvolumes detected by the hypoxia tracer ^{18}F-fluoromisonidazole (FMISO). Theoretical IMRT plans were designed for 10 patients, giving 70 Gy to the FDG PET/CT GTV and a boost to a total dose of 84 Gy to the hypoxic subvolumes inside the GTV as defined by FMISO-PET. The study showed that a dose escalation plan could be achieved in all 10 patients without exceeding the normal tissue tolerances. Lee and colleagues also attempted to boost the hypoxic subvolume to 105 Gy in 2 patients, and were successful in one patient with a relatively small hypoxia subvolume. Lin and colleagues,[58] in the same group, also performed a feasibility study for dose escalation using FMISO-PET, and evaluated the reproducibility of the FMISO-PET scan by obtaining 2 scans separated by 3 days before radiotherapy. When comparing the serial FMISO-PET scans, they found that the hypoxic volume had significantly changed in 4 of 7 patients, which could have compromised the planned boost dose. The inconsistency in the hypoxic volume between two scans can be attributed to a variety of causes, such as technical issues, but tumor hypoxia is not a static process and can change over time, especially after treatment when reoxygenation occurs. Further studies are necessary to reveal the implication for subvolume delineation using hypoxia tracers.

These studies demonstrate the feasibility of designing subvolumes based on radiopharmaceuticals other than FDG. However, further clinical trials are necessary to determine whether dose escalation to the hypoxic regions could lead to improved local control of the disease.

SUMMARY

FDG-PET imaging is being used more frequently by radiation oncologists for radiation treatment planning. PET is a powerful tool that provides metabolic/biologic data that can aid the oncologist in staging, treatment planning, and patient management. New gradient and adaptive threshold algorithms appear promising with regard to segmentation, and may reduce variability among radiation oncologists. We may find that the optimal segmentation method may vary according to subsite (eg, glottis, base of tongue). Studies in dose escalation to PET volumes will hopefully lead to improved local control of tumor, although randomized trials comparing dose escalation to conventional IMRT are needed. Finally, advances in PET and CT technology will hopefully lead to continued improvements in resolution, and new radiotracers will enable us to better refine the specific metabolic process in tumors for target delineation.

REFERENCES

1. Jemal A, Siegel R, Ward E, et al. Cancer statistics, 2009. CA Cancer J Clin 2009;59:225–49.
2. Adelstein DL, Li Y, Adams GL, et al. An intergroup phase III comparison of standard radiation and two schedules of concurrent chemoradiotherapy in patients with unresectable squamous cell head and neck cancer. J Clin Oncol 2003;21:92–8.
3. Forastiere AA, Goepfert H, Maor M, et al. Concurrent chemotherapy and radiotherapy for organ preservation in advanced laryngeal cancer. N Engl J Med 2003;329:2091–8.
4. Al-Sarraf M, LeBlanc M, Giri PG, et al. Chemoradiotherapy versus radiotherapy in patients with advanced nasopharyngeal cancer: phase III randomized Intergroup study 0099. J Clin Oncol 1998;16:1310–7.
5. Cooper JS, Pajak TF, Forastiere AA, et al. Postoperative concurrent radiotherapy and chemotherapy for high-risk squamous-cell carcinoma of the head and neck. N Engl J Med 2004;350:1937–44.
6. Bernier J, Domenge C, Ozsahim M, et al. Postoperative irradiation with or without concomitant chemotherapy for locally advanced head and neck cancer. N Engl J Med 2004;350:1945–52.
7. Mell L, Mehrotra A, Mundt A. Intensity-modulated radiation therapy use in the US, 2004. Cancer 2005;104:1296–303.
8. Lee N, Puri D, Blanco A, et al. Intensity-modulated radiation therapy in head and neck cancers: an update. Head Neck 2007;29:387–400.
9. Gregoire V, De Neve W, Eisbruch A, et al. Intensity-modulated radiation therapy for head and neck carcinoma. Oncologist 2007;12:555–64.
10. Chao KS, Deasy J, Markman J, et al. A prospective study of salivary function sparing in patients with head-and-neck cancers receiving intensity-modulated or three-dimensional radiation therapy: initial results. Int J Radiat Oncol Biol Phys 2001;49:907–16.
11. Lin A, Kim HM, Terrell J, et al. Quality of life after parotid-sparing IMRT for head-and-neck cancer: a prospective longitudinal study. Int J Radiat Oncol Biol Phys 2003;57:61–70.

12. Yao M, Karnell LH, Funk GF, et al. Health-related quality-of-life outcomes following IMRT versus conventional radiotherapy for oropharyngeal squamous cell carcinoma. Int J Radiat Oncol Biol Phys 2007;69:1354–60.

13. Roh J, Yeo N, Kim JS, et al. Utility of 2-[18F] fluoro-2-deoxy-D-glucose positron emission tomography and positron emission tomography/computed tomography imaging in the preoperative staging of head and neck squamous cell carcinoma. Oral Oncology 2007;43:887–93.

14. Ng S, Yen T, Liao C, et al. 18F-FDG PET and CT/MRI in oral cavity squamous cell carcinoma: a prospective study of 124 patients with histologic correlation. J Nucl Med 2005;46:1136–43.

15. Al-Ibraheem A, Buck A, Krause BJ, et al. Clinical applications of FDG PET and PET/CT in head and neck cancer. J Oncol 2009;2009:208725.

16. McCollum AD, Burrell S, Haddad R, et al. Positron emission tomography with 18F-fluorodeoxyglucose to predict pathologic response after induction chemotherapy and definitive chemoradiotherapy in head and neck cancer. Head Neck 2004;26:890–6.

17. Yen R, Chen TH, Ting L, et al. Early restaging whole-body 18F-FDG PET during induction chemotherapy predicts clinical outcome in patients with locoregionally advanced nasopharyngeal carcinoma. Eur J Nucl Med Mol Imaging 2005;32:1152–9.

18. Yao M, Smith R, Hoffman H, et al. Clinical significance of postradiotherapy 18F-fluorodeoxyglucose positron emission tomography imaging in management of head-and-neck cancer-a long term outcome report. Int J Radiat Oncol Biol Phys 2009;74:9–14.

19. Simpson DR, Lawson JD, Nath SK, et al. Utilization of advanced imaging technologies for target delineation in radiation oncology. J Am Coll Radiol 2009;6:876–83.

20. Schwartz D, Ford EC, Rajendran J, et al. FDG-PET/CT-guided intensity modulated head and neck radiotherapy: a pilot investigation. Head Neck 2005;27:478–87.

21. Mattes D, Haynor D, Vesselle, et al. PET-CT image registration in the chest using free-form deformations. IEEE Trans Med Imaging 2003;22:120–8.

22. Vogel WV, Schinagl DA, Van Dalen JA, et al. Validated image fusion of dedicated PET and CT for external beam radiation and therapy in the head and neck area. Q J Nucl Med Mol Imaging 2008; 52:74–83.

23. Ireland R, Dyker K, Barber D, et al. Nonrigid image registration for head and neck cancer radiotherapy treatment planning with PET/CT. Int J Radiat Oncol Biol Phys 2007;68:952–7.

24. Hwang AB, Bacharach SL, Yom SS, et al. Can positron emission tomography (PET) or PET/computed tomography (CT) acquired in a nontreatment position be accurately registered to a head-and-neck

25. Park SB, Rhee FC, Monroe JI, et al. Spatial weighted mutual information for image registration in image guided radiation therapy. Med Phys 2010;37: 4590–601.

26. Ciernik IF, Dizendorf E, Baumert BG, et al. Radiation treatment planning with an integrated positron emission and computer tomography (PET/CT): a feasibility study. Int J Radiat Oncol Biol Phys 2003;57:853–63.

27. Paulino AC, Koshy M, Howell R, et al. Comparison of CT- and FDG-PET-defined gross tumor volume in intensity-modulated radiotherapy for head-and-neck cancer. Int J Radiat Oncol Biol Phys 2005;61: 1385–92.

28. Deantonio L, Beldì D, Gambaro G, et al. FDG-PET/CT imaging for staging and radiotherapy treatment planning of head and neck carcinoma. Radiat Oncol 2008;3:29.

29. Guido A, Fuccio L, Rombi B, et al. Combined 18F-FDG-PET/CT imaging in radiotherapy target delineation for head-and-neck cancer. Int J Radiat Oncol Biol Phys 2009;73:759–63.

30. Scarfone C, Lavely WC, Cmelak AJ, et al. Prospective feasibility trial of radiotherapy target definition for head and neck cancer using 3-dimensional PET and CT imaging. J Nucl Med 2004;45:543–52.

31. El-Bassiouni M, Ciernik IF, Davis JB, et al. [18FDG] PET-CT-based intensity-modulated radiotherapy treatment planning of head and neck cancer. Int J Radiat Oncol Biol Phys 2007;69:286–93.

32. Henriques de Figueiredo B, Barret O, Demeaux H, et al. Comparison between CT- and FDG-PET-defined target volumes for radiotherapy planning in head-and-neck cancers. Radiother Oncol 2009;93:479–82.

33. Wang D, Schultz CJ, Jursinic PA, et al. Initial experience of FDG-PET/CT guided IMRT of head-and-neck carcinoma. Int J Radiat Oncol Biol Phys 2006;65:143–51.

34. Heron DE, Andrade RS, Flickinger J, et al. Hybrid PET-CT simulation for radiation treatment planning in head-and-neck cancers: a brief technical report. Int J Radiat Oncol Biol Phys 2004;60:1419–24.

35. Schinagl DA, Vogel WV, Hoffmann AL, et al. Comparison of five segmentation tools for 18F-fluoro-deoxy-glucose-positron emission tomography-based target volume definition in head and neck cancer. Int J Radiat Oncol Biol Phys 2007;69:1282–9.

36. Greco C, Nehmeh SA, Schöder H, et al. Evaluation of different methods of 18F-FDG-PET target volume delineation in the radiotherapy of head and neck cancer. Am J Clin Oncol 2008;31:439–45.

37. Daisne J, Sibomana M, Bol A, et al. Tri-dimensional automatic segmentation of PET volumes based on measured source-to-background ratios: influence of reconstruction algorithms. Radiother Oncol 2003; 69:247–50.

38. Adams R, Bischof L. Seeded region growing. IEEE Trans Pattern Anal Mach Intell 1994;16:641–7.

39. Hsu PK, Huang HC, Hsieh CC, et al. Effect of formalin fixation on tumor size determination in stage I non-small cell lung cancer. Ann Thorac Surg 2007; 84:1825–9.

40. Burri RJ, Rangaswamy B, Kostakoglu L, et al. Correlation of positron emission tomography standard uptake value and pathologic specimen size in cancer of the head and neck. Int J Radiat Oncol Biol Phys 2008;71:682–8.

41. Daisne JF, Duprez T, Weynand B, et al. Tumor volume in pharyngolaryngeal squamous cell carcinoma: comparison at CT, MR imaging, and FDG PET and validation with surgical specimen. Radiology 2004;233:93–100.

42. Seitz O, Chambron-Pinho N, Middendorp M, et al. ^{18}F-Fluorodeoxyglucose-PET/CT to evaluate tumor, nodal disease, and gross tumor volume of oropharyngeal and oral cavity cancer: comparison with MR imaging and validation with surgical specimen. Neuroradiology 2009;51:677–86.

43. Geets X, Lee JA, Bol A, et al. A gradient-based method for segmenting FDG-PET images: methodology and validation. Eur J Nucl Med Mol Imaging 2007;34:1427–38.

44. Vernon MR, Maheshwari M, Schultz CJ, et al. Clinical outcomes of patients receiving integrated PET/CT-guided radiotherapy for head and neck carcinoma. Int J Radiat Oncol Biol Phys 2008;70:678–84.

45. Yao M, Dornfeld KJ, Buatti JM, et al. Intensity-modulated radiation treatment for head-and-neck squamous cell carcinoma–the University of Iowa experience. Int J Radiat Oncol Biol Phys 2005;63:410–21.

46. Chao KS, Ozyigit G, Tran BN, et al. Patterns of failure in patients receiving definitive and postoperative IMRT for head-and-neck cancer. Int J Radiat Oncol Biol Phys 2003;55:312–21.

47. Dawson LA, Anzai Y, Marsh L, et al. Patterns of local-regional recurrence following parotid-sparing conformal and segmental intensity-modulated radiotherapy for head and neck cancer. Int J Radiat Oncol Biol Phys 2000;46:1117–26.

48. Mees G, Dierckx R, Vangestel C, et al. Molecular imaging of hypoxia with radiolabelled agents. Eur J Nucl Med Mol Imaging 2009;36:1674–86.

49. Pugachev A, Ruan S, Carlin S, et al. Dependence of FDG uptake on tumor microenvironment. Int J Radiat Oncol Biol Phys 2005;62:545–53.

50. Allal AS, Slosman DO, Kebdani T, et al. Prediction of outcome in head-and-neck cancer patients using the standardized uptake value of 2-[^{18}F]fluoro-2-deoxy-D-glucose. Int J Radiat Oncol Biol Phys 2004;59:1295–300.

51. Machtay M, Natwa M, Andrel J, et al. Pretreatment FDG-PET standardized uptake value as a prognostic factor for outcome in head and neck cancer. Head Neck 2009;31:195–201.

52. Yao M, Lu M, Savvides P, et al. The prognostic significance of pretreatment SUV in head-and-neck squamous cell carcinoma treated with IMRT. Int J Radiat Oncol Biol Phys 2009;75:S17.

53. Madani I, Duthoy W, Derie C, et al. Positron emission tomography-guided, focal-dose escalation using intensity-modulated radiotherapy for head and neck cancer. Int J Radiat Oncol Biol Phys 2007;68: 126–35.

54. Geets X, Daisne JF, Gregoire V, et al. Role of 11-C-methionine positron emission tomography for the delineation of the tumor volume in pharyngolaryngeal squamous cell carcinoma: comparison with FDG-PET and CT. Radiother Oncol 2004;71:267–73.

55. Chao KS, Bosch WR, Mutic S, et al. A novel approach to overcome hypoxic tumor resistance: Cu-ATSM-guided intensity-modulated radiation therapy. Int J Radiat Oncol Biol Phys 2001;49: 1171–82.

56. Grosu AL, Souvatzoglou M, Röper B, et al. Hypoxia imaging with FAZA-PET and theoretical considerations with regard to dose painting for individualization of radiotherapy in patients with head and neck cancer. Int J Radiat Oncol Biol Phys 2007;69:541–51.

57. Lee N, Mechalakos JG, Nehmeh S, et al. Fluorine-18-labeled fluoromisonidazole positron emission and computed tomography-guided intensity-modulated radiotherapy for head-and-neck cancer: a feasibility study. Int J Radiat Oncol Biol Phys 2008;70:2–13.

58. Lin Z, Mechalakos JG, Nehmeh S, et al. The influence of changes in tumor hypoxia on dose-painting treatment planes based on ^{18}F-FMISO positron emission tomography. Int J Radiat Oncol Biol Phys 2008;70: 1219–28.

PET–Computed Tomography for Radiation Treatment Planning of Lymphoma and Hematologic Malignancies

Stephanie A. Terezakis, MD[a], Joachim Yahalom, MD[b],*

KEYWORDS

- FDG-PET • Radiation treatment • Lymphoma
- Hematologic malignancy

Metabolically active tumor cells are functionally distinct because of their increased glycolytic activity relative to normal cells. Whole-body imaging using PET uses the radiolabeled glucose analogue, fludeoxyglucose F 18 (FDG), which is preferentially taken up by malignant cells. Tumor cells are characterized by the upregulation of glucose transport as well as hexokinase activity. The phosphorylation of hexokinase leads to the accumulation of FDG in malignant relative to nonmalignant cells. PET imaging complements computed tomographic (CT) scan anatomic information by localizing metabolically active cells within the anatomic tumor volume. FDG uptake is seen not only in malignant processes but also in inflammatory and infectious processes. Nevertheless, the sensitivity and specificity of PET relative to CT and magnetic resonance (MR) imaging is increased for malignancies, such as lymphoma, and thus these techniques play a critical role in diagnostic workup and treatment response evaluation. As a result of the utility of PET in the evaluation of lymphoma, interest in incorporating PET into radiation planning has grown.[1–7]

Radiation oncology has made substantial progress in technology with the development of conformal radiation treatment techniques, such as intensity-modulated radiotherapy, stereotactic radiotherapy, and stereotactic radiosurgery. These systems deliver radiation with high precision and leave little room for errors in targeting the tumor (**Fig. 1**). Diagnostic imaging is used to aid the radiation oncologist in target volume definition (**Fig. 2**). Three-dimensional tumor volumes are routinely developed using CT scan treatment planning or simulation based on standard definitions defined by the International Commission on Radiation Units and Measurements, ICRU50. Lymphoma disease extent is assessed with physical examination; tissue biopsy, including bone marrow biopsy; and imaging modalities. Although CT provides important anatomic definition, it has its limitations. Small-volume nodal disease that can have significant implications on radiation treatment field design can be missed (**Fig. 3**). Residual masses after chemotherapy that may represent scar tissue can also be difficult to interpret in the absence of functional imaging. PET contributes

a Department of Radiation Oncology and Molecular Radiation Sciences, Johns Hopkins School of Medicine, Weinberg Comprehensive Cancer Center, 401 North Broadway Suite 1440, Baltimore, MD 21231, USA
b Department of Radiation Oncology, Memorial Sloan-Kettering Cancer Center, 1275 York Avenue, New York, NY 10022, USA
* Corresponding author.
E-mail address: yahalomj@mskcc.org

PET Clin 6 (2011) 165–175
doi:10.1016/j.cpet.2011.03.003

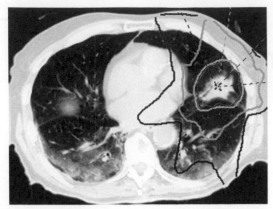

Fig. 1. Example of radiation plan created using intensity-modulated radiotherapy (IMRT) in a patient who presented with a peripheral lung mass contoured on a CT treatment-planning scan. With IMRT, a concave dose distribution can be accomplished to deliver prescription dose to the tumor volume while protecting normal structures, including surrounding normal lung. The surrounding multicolored lines represent isodose distributions. Each color represents a percentage of the prescribed dose received by the given volume encompassed within the curve. Precision in target volume delineation is essential when the radiation dose is prescribed with highly conformal techniques.

complementary information and can aid in disease assessment for the purpose of delineating anatomic areas at risk. Therefore, PET has been integrated into radiation treatment planning and contributes functional information to the design of the tumor volume to help create a biologic target volume (BTV). The BTV is a concept proposed by Ling and colleagues[8] that takes into account the tumor as depicted on functional imaging, such as PET.

Although radiation treatment is integral to the management of lymphoma, extended fields (extended field radiotherapy [EFRT]) are no longer commonly treated because of significant normal-tissue exposure. Most patients with early-stage lymphoma are now treated with combined-modality therapy using chemotherapy followed by involved field radiation therapy (IFRT), which includes the involved site and immediately adjacent lymph node regions in the treatment field.[9] Thus, lymphoma radiation treatment field design has undergone an evolution from EFRT to IFRT.[9] Involved node radiotherapy (INRT) shrinks fields further so that only the involved lymph nodes with a margin is included in the radiation treatment field. INRT is now under active investigation. Initial studies suggest that relapse rates with INRT are equivalent to those with IFRT and EFRT for patients

with early-stage Hodgkin disease (HD) and early-stage follicular lymphoma.[10,11] However, the application of INRT and conformal techniques requires a higher level of precision in identifying involved disease because of the greater potential for a marginal miss.

FDG-PET RADIATION PLANNING FOR LYMPHOMA

PET scan has become an integral aspect of the diagnostic workup for lymphoma because its utility in staging has been demonstrated in multiple studies.[12–18] Stumpe and colleagues[19] demonstrated a specificity of 96% for PET compared with 41% for the staging of patients with HD and a specificity of 100% compared with 67% for patients with non-Hodgkin lymphoma (NHL). However, FDG avidity varies widely depending on lymphoma subtype. Aggressive NHLs, such as diffuse large B cell lymphoma, and HD are more likely to be FDG avid than low-grade NHLs, such as follicular and marginal zone lymphomas.[15,20–23] FDG avidity in low-grade lymphomas can also be inconsistent, and thus, PET may not be as useful for target delineation in these cases in which FDG distribution could be variable.[12,24–26] However, staging conclusions can sometimes be difficult to derive because it is often not feasible to obtain pathologic proof of lymphoma at each FDG-avid site, given the systemic nature of the disease. Because inflammation, reactivity, and infection can also cause uptake on PET, the physician must use all available clinical information, including physical examination, imaging, and pathology, to delineate the target in the absence of pathologic confirmation.

Given the usefulness of PET in defining disease extent, it has been increasingly incorporated into radiotherapy planning to help in the definition of radiation treatment fields. An FDG-PET scan obtained in a nuclear medicine department can be coregistered to a CT treatment-planning scan obtained in a radiation oncology department. The patient should be placed in the treatment-planning position using an appropriate individualized immobilization device for the PET scan as well as for the CT treatment-planning scan. The PET scan is then transferred and fused with the CT treatment-planning scan. However, if the patient's position varies between the 2 independently performed scans, it may be more difficult to confidently delineate the target. Dedicated PET/CT scanners for simulation can minimize this error by acquiring both the PET and CT scans in the same session so that the scans can be immediately coregistered for radiation planning. For

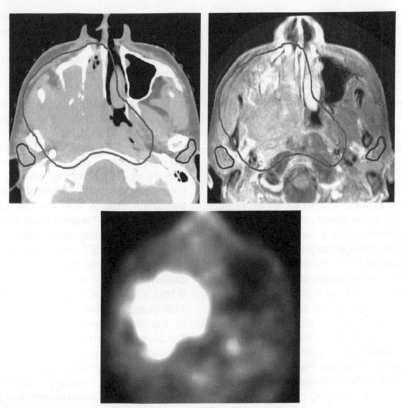

Fig. 2. Fusion of CT, PET, and MRI allows the advantages of each modality to be used in delineating the GTV (*dark blue contour*) for this patient with nasal natural killer/T-cell lymphoma. The red contour represents the bilateral parotid glands and aqua contour represents the brainstem.

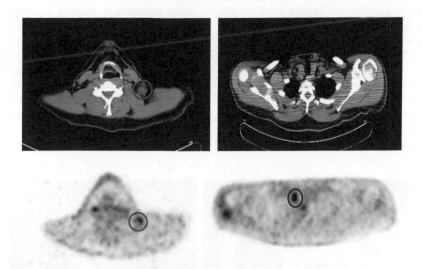

Fig. 3. This patient initially presented with an enlarged left supraclavicular node, which was biopsied and consistent with diffuse large B cell lymphoma (DLBCL). PET scan was subsequently performed and identified an FDG-avid site on the contralateral neck, which localized to what appeared as a thyroid nodule on CT scan. Because of the concern for FDG avidity, the contralateral neck was biopsied and DLBCL was identified. Without PET, the contralateral neck disease would not have been identified and the patient would have received consolidative radiation to an incorrect unilateral neck involved field. The blue contour represents biopsy-proven DLBCL in the left neck and the purple contour represents biopsy-proven DLBCL in the right neck.

example, the head and neck is a particularly difficult treatment site to accurately coregister PET and CT because of the flexibility of the neck, which can make it difficult to register the upper and lower neck simultaneously.[27–29] FDG distribution in the head and neck region is also considered more complex than that in other treatment sites because of the presence of normal structures with nonpathologic FDG uptake, and thus, an accurate fusion can be invaluable.

Although the use of PET in radiation planning for lymphomas has a strong rationale, PET radiation planning was first studied in non–small cell lung cancer (NSCLC) and head and neck cancer. Based on extensive study in the literature of PET planning for these malignancies, it is evident that the integration of PET can change staging, management, and target volumes.[30–39] Several prospective studies have been performed in NSCLC. In the first prospective analysis of radiotherapy planning using PET/CT fusion by Giraud and colleagues,[33] the gross tumor volume (GTV) was altered in 5 of 12 patients as a result of findings identified on PET. Mah and colleagues[36] performed a similar study prospectively analyzing the GTV and planning target volume (PTV) delineated on CT alone compared with PET imaging in 30 patients. Patients in this study had tumors that were not easily defined on CT scan. With the addition of PET, the treatment intent was altered in 30% of patients from definitive to palliative. In addition, the GTV was altered to include PET-identified regional (within 5 cm) lymph nodes in 5 of 23 patients who received definitive therapy. This study also specifically examined interobserver variability in delineating the GTV and PTV and concluded that the addition of PET significantly reduced variability in treatment volume contouring. In a prospective study of 26 patients performed by Bradley and colleagues,[38] 8 patients were upstaged with PET and 2 received palliative radiation because of metastatic disease identified using PET. The radiation treatment volume was altered in 58% of patients; the GTV decreased in 3 patients and increased in 11 patients.

PET may have a pertinent role in cases in which tumor is difficult to differentiate from atelectasis, which may be particularly useful for mediastinal lymphomas (Fig. 4). With the exclusion of atelectasis, reduction in radiation treatment field size may be possible using the additional information provided by PET. Although studies focusing on lymphoma have not yet explored this possible benefit of PET planning, analyses published on lung cancer have demonstrated reduction in treatment volume with the use of PET in cases with atelectasis. Treatment volumes were contoured in patients diagnosed with locally advanced NSCLC using PET alone compared with CT in a study by Nestle and colleagues.[31] Of the 12 patients in whom the treatment volume changed, 9 had a reduction in volume with the exclusion of atelectasis, a distinction aided by the use of PET at the time of target delineation. A decrease in the size of the irradiation field could substantially reduce toxicity, particularly, if atelectasis, associated with presumably normal lung, is excluded. Therefore, PET radiation planning may have particular utility in distinguishing between tumor and associated atelectasis both for obtaining accuracy in target volume delineation as well as for minimizing the irradiation of normal tissues.[31]

The effect of PET on the design of the radiation target volume for head and neck cancer has been reported in several studies. Nishioka and colleagues[28] specifically analyzed patients with oropharyngeal and nasopharyngeal primary tumors. In most patients (90%), the primary lesion GTV was unchanged. However, for 2 patients, the GTV changed significantly. The investigators also reported that the absence of FDG activity allowed the sparing of normal structures. Rahn and colleagues[40] also integrated PET scan into radiation planning with CT, MR imaging, and ultrasonography

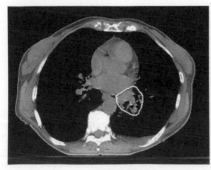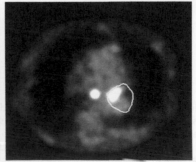

Fig. 4. Use of PET/CT fusion for GTV delineation (*yellow contour*); in this case, the FDG-avid lesion is apparent in the mediastinum, and the PET information aids in the delineation of tumor from normal structures.

in 34 patients with squamous cell cancer of the head and neck. FDG-PET–identified lymph node metastases in a large number of patients, leading to changes in radiation field and dose. Overall, a significant change in the radiation treatment plan occurred in 15 of 34 patients with primary and recurrent diseases. Ciernik and colleagues[39] also studied 12 patients with head and neck cancer using the integrated PET/CT system. When comparing the GTV contoured using PET/CT with that using CT alone, the GTV increased by 25% or more in 17% of cases and decreased by more than 25% in 33% of patients, although MR imaging was not used in this study.

A growing body of literature specifically examines the effect of FDG-PET in radiation treatment planning of patients with lymphoma.[3–6,41,42] Initial studies have suggested that the integration of PET at the time of simulation can result in a change in management, target volume, and doses to normal structures. Lee and colleagues[7] retrospectively studied PET radiation planning in 15 patients with thoracic lymphoma by manually registering PET and CT scans. The investigators analyzed 10 PET scans with positive results; in 4 of 10 patients, the difference in lateral extension of the treatment field was greater than 3 cm. In 3 of these cases, the PET-defined GTV was smaller than the GTV as defined on CT scan. In this analysis, the inferior extent of the CT-based treatment fields was significantly greater than PET-based treatment fields in 2 patients. Phantom planning with lead blocking led to a decrease of 50% in lung dose in these patients. This study demonstrated the potential for reduction in normal tissue doses with the integration of PET in select cases.

In the study by Lee and colleagues,[7] the PET-defined GTV likely did not include apparent CT scan abnormalities. Lymphoma radiation treatment

fields must be cautiously designed in the clinical scenario in which a CT scan abnormality is noted in the absence of FDG avidity. Picardi and colleagues[43] reported on 260 patients with bulky HD who were treated with chemotherapy, of whom 160 achieved a negative PET scan result. Patients with a negative PET scan result were then randomized to either receive further treatment with radiation or undergo observation. Histologic evaluation demonstrated that 14% of patients in the chemotherapy-alone arm had malignant disease compared with 4% of patients in the radiation arm. All patients who relapsed in the chemotherapy arm had persistent disease within the bulky or contiguous nodal region. Thus, patients with a negative PET scan result but a residual CT abnormality may still be at risk for relapse because of the presence of microscopic disease. As a result, the authors include the extent of the CT abnormality even in sites in which the PET scan result is negative because there is an absence of studies that correlate pathology with extent of PET scan positivity specifically in lymphoma. Therefore, the authors continue to recommend the inclusion of both CT and PET abnormalities in the target volume.

Hutchings and colleagues[5] studied 30 patients with early-stage HD who received a staging FDG-PET/CT. A short course of doxorubicin hydrochloride (Adriamycin), bleomycin, vinblastine, and dacarbazine was delivered before radiation treatment. IFRT planning was initially performed using a CT treatment-planning scan alone, but treatment in patients was then planned using contours delineated on PET/CT. The integration of FDG-PET information would have resulted in an increase in the treated volume in 7 patients in whom FDG-avid areas were identified outside the treated volume (**Fig. 5**). In these patients, the volume receiving 90% of the prescription dose

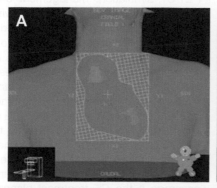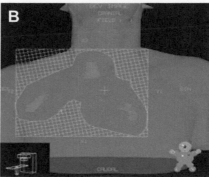

Fig. 5. The patient presented with stage IIA disease and had a PET-positive focus in the right axilla, which had not been identified on the staging CT. The projections of the different planning treatment volumes are shown. (*A*) CT radiation planning. (*B*) PET/CT radiation planning. (*From* Hutchings M, Loft A, Hansen M, et al. Clinical impact of FDG-PET/CT in the planning of radiotherapy for early-stage Hodgkin lymphoma. Eur J Hematol 2007;78:210; with permission.)

was increased by 8% to 87%. A decrease in the treated volume would have occurred in 2 patients. As Hutchings and colleagues noted, radiation oncologists are reluctant to reduce the size of a treatment field targeting an FDG-negative mass unless the CT scan abnormality was truly indeterminate. Realizing that both imaging modalities do not have a sensitivity or specificity of 100%, the treatment volume should encompass suspicious abnormalities on both CT and PET scans, which potentially results in overall larger volumes using PET/CT than those on the CT scan alone.

A study by Dizendorf and colleagues[3] reviewed 202 consecutive patients with various malignancies, of whom 24 were diagnosed with lymphoma, who underwent FDG-PET scan for radiation planning. Because of information acquired using PET, management strategy was altered in 21% of patients and a change in target volume was implemented in 13% of patients with lymphoma. Brianzoni and colleagues[41] also studied 28 patients, of whom 4 presented with NHL. FDG-PET scan was acquired in all patients and registered to CT images for radiation planning. The clinical target volume (CTV) was not altered in any patient, but radiation treatment did not proceed in 1 patient because of findings on PET.

Girinsky and colleagues[4] also specifically studied patients with early-stage HD and addressed the challenge of contouring a prechemotherapy volume on a postchemotherapy CT-planning scan. Pretreatment CT and FDG-PET scans were performed in the treatment position and were coregistered with a postchemotherapy CT simulation-planning scan. FDG-PET helped to delineate lymph nodes that were otherwise undetectable on CT scan in 36% of patients. Hence, prechemotherapy FDG-PET scans can identify lymph node sites that require consolidative radiation. As a result, the incorporation of PET scan may be crucial in the accurate design of INRT fields, which require the precise identification of involved sites of disease. The current European Organization for Research and Treatment of Cancer/Groupe d'Etudes des Lymphomes de l'Adulte (EORTC-GELA) guidelines for the design of INRT fields recommend routine use of prechemotherapy FDG-PET scans, which are performed in the treatment position with radiation-specific immobilization devices.[44]

A recent large-scale prospective multicenter study was published by Pommier and colleagues[45] that reported the effect of preradiation PET scan on management strategy and radiation planning for 137 patients in 11 centers with early-stage HD. The radiation plan was initially created with the CT information alone and then modified based on the addition of the PET acquired. All patients except one received chemotherapy before radiation. With the integration of PET, there was a change in radiation treatment dose, volume, or dosimetric plan in 12.9% of patients. Radiation was canceled in 4.8% of patients. When a prechemotherapy PET scan was obtained, the concordance between preradiotherapy and postradiotherapy plans was high. Overall, the concordance between treatment strategy before and after preradiotherapy PET was 82.3%. Therefore, information garnered from a preradiation PET scan can lead to significant changes in management as well as radiation treatment volume.

In most patients studied in the previously discussed analyses, IFRT is given after a complete response to chemotherapy. Therefore, in these cases, the postchemotherapy PET scan result is negative, and the involved field is designed using anatomic information derived from CT scan and the prechemotherapy PET scan. However, there is a subset of patients who are referred for radiation with positive PET scan results at the time of treatment. These patients include those referred for primary treatment with radiation alone (ie, patients with mucosa-associated lymphoid tissue or follicular lymphoma), partial responders to chemotherapy who cannot receive additional systemic therapy, or patients with relapsed/refractory disease referred for IFRT in the setting of high-dose salvage treatment. In these cases, PET results may be positive at the time of radiotherapy and thus may be helpful in providing additional functional information (**Fig. 6**).

Findings at the time of simulation were described in a cohort of patients with hematologic malignancies by Terezakis and colleagues.[6] In this study, 29 patients with positive PET scan results at the time of treatment planning were identified. Because of unexpected findings at the time of PET/CT simulation, management changed in 2 patients who did not proceed with radiation because of findings of advanced disease. The addition of PET changed the volume in 23 of 32 treatment sites (72%). The PTV was increased in 15 sites (47%) and reduced in 8 sites (25%). The treatment in all patients was replanned in this study using CT alone and PET volumes. The D95 and V95 decreased by more than 5% in 6 patients when the CT-based plan was used to cover the PET volume. Therefore, if it is assumed that PET-positive sites include active disease, 6 patients would not have had adequate target volume coverage if the CT treatment-planning scan information were used without the information derived from PET. Although study numbers were small, it was apparent that patients with aggressive lymphoma histologic subtypes (ie, atypical

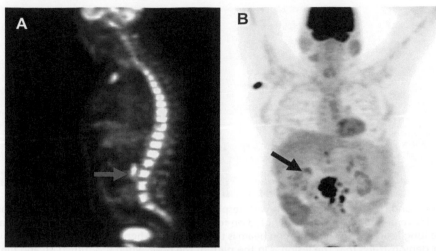

Fig. 6. A patient with atypical Burkitt-like lymphoma presented for simulation. A PET, at the time of simulation, unexpectedly identified progression of disease in para-aortic and pelvic nodes even though the patient had a recent PET scan 3 weeks before simulation. (*A*) Presimulation PET scan (*arrow*). (*B*) Postsimulation PET scan (*arrow*).

Burkitt-like lymphoma) were most likely to have significant changes in target volume and management, suggesting that PET may play its greatest role in the treatment planning of these patients.

TECHNICAL CONSIDERATIONS

There are several technical considerations, including windowing level, image resolution, and patient motion, that must be taken into account to accurately coregister and interpret PET and CT images for the purpose of tumor volume definition.[39,46] Patients are specifically positioned for treatment planning, using site-specific immobilization for radiation planning during simulation. CT simulation is now considered standard in radiation oncology departments across the country. A dialogue between radiation oncology and nuclear medicine must occur for patients to undergo PET scan in the treatment position, particularly, if an immobilization device is used. Geometric alignment results in a more accurate fusion between PET and CT scans. It is a frequent occurrence that the patient is not in an acceptable position for radiation treatment when a PET scan is performed for staging or response assessment workup. Although there are methods for fusing PET and CT scans, which are separately acquired, one image may have to be deformed to fuse with the other image, which could lead to inaccuracies.[28,47–50] In rapidly proliferating malignancies, a recent PET should also be acquired if it is used for radiotherapy-planning purposes because the extent of disease may change in a short period.[6]

Although several studies have demonstrated a reduction in interobserver variability with the use of PET/CT for treatment planning, there are challenges in defining target volumes with PET.[36] Because of the resolution of PET, the size of PET-detected lesions is generally larger than 1 cm, whereas CT scan can detect lesions that are approximately 5 mm.[34,49,51–53] The definition of the borders of the lesion can be variable depending on the windowing level and contrast between the tumor and the background. The CT component of the PET fusion can provide anatomic data to aid in target volume definition when lesions appear "fuzzy." To properly define the tumor volume with the use of PET fusion, close clinical correlation must be used and PET interpretation must be performed with a nuclear medicine physician.

To limit the variability in contouring with the use of PET, a protocol used to acquire the PET must be implemented consistently. A reliable methodology used to fuse the PET with the CT at the time of planning must also exist. The PET and CT must be properly coregistered, and the window level used for contouring should be defined in conjunction with nuclear medicine. To define the edge of the GTV, a threshold is often chosen by using either a cutoff based on absolute standardized uptake value (SUV) or a fixed percentage intensity level relative to the maximum activity in the lesion. An SUV threshold used to define malignant versus benign tissues remains unknown. Both cutoff approaches are imperfect with the potential for inaccuracies in reproducibility and volume estimation.[27,36,38,39,54–57]

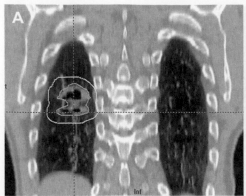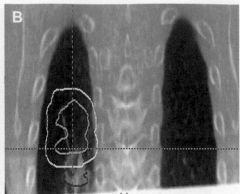

Fig. 7. Evaluation and treatment of a patient with respiratory gating with visualization of respiratory motion of the target. (*A*) Movement of the lung lesion noted on four-dimensional CT scan at the time of simulation. (*B*) The location of the lung lesion when the radiation beam is turned on and when the radiation beam is turned off. The green contour demonstrates that the lesion is in the path of the beam when it is turned on and the lesion is out of the path of the beam when the beam is turned off. The yellow contour represents the PTV.

Tumors are also subject to movement. PET is generally performed over multiple respiratory cycles, and therefore, the image obtained represents the tumor's position throughout the entire respiratory cycle. As a result, the PET-defined volume may be larger than that by CT.[47,48,58] Respiratory gating can be used to trigger the radiation beam to turn on only during a specified portions of the breathing cycle (**Fig. 7**).[59] External markers on the body surface can serve as the signal to indicate the phases of the breathing cycle and trigger the beam. Four-dimensional gated PET/CT protocols can be timed with the patient's respiratory cycle to potentially decrease the size of the target volume by accounting for respiratory motion.[60–63] Scan preparation factors, such as time between tracer injection and scanning, patient blood glucose level, lesion size, and room temperature, can affect the measurement of FDG uptake.

Studies have demonstrated that FDG-PET can be useful in identifying tumor volumes, reducing interobserver variability, and distinguishing disease from atelectasis. However, clinical correlation and consultation with an expert nuclear medicine physician is necessary to interpret PET results for tumor volume contouring. Ultimately, precise delineation of the CTV from normal structures still remains challenging despite the additional information that can be provided by PET.

SUMMARY

FDG-PET is an extremely useful tool for staging and response assessment in multiple malignancies. The growing importance of this technique in radiation treatment planning has also been

demonstrated in multiple studies. However, there are many potential pitfalls of PET, particularly in radiation planning, and radiation oncologists must be mindful of the complexities of PET before adapting it for routine use. Close collaboration with nuclear medicine is essential to appropriately interpret PET findings for the design of radiation treatment volumes. Ultimately, long-term clinical outcomes are needed to determine the effect of PET in radiation planning.

REFERENCES

1. Dwamena BA, Sonnad SS, Angobaldo JO, et al. Metastases from non-small cell lung cancer: mediastinal staging in the 1990s—meta-analytic comparison of PET and CT. Radiology 1999;213(2):530–6.
2. Fletcher JW, Djulbegovic B, Soares HP, et al. Recommendations on the use of 18F-FDG PET in oncology. J Nucl Med 2008;49(3):480–508.
3. Dizendorf EV, Baumert BG, von Schulthess GK, et al. Impact of whole-body 18F-FDG PET on staging and managing patients for radiation therapy. J Nucl Med 2003;44(1):24–9.
4. Girinsky T, Ghalibafian M, Bonniaud G, et al. Is FDG-PET scan in patients with early stage Hodgkin lymphoma of any value in the implementation of the involved-node radiotherapy concept and dose painting? Radiother Oncol 2007;85(2):178–86.
5. Hutchings M, Loft A, Hansen M, et al. Clinical impact of FDG-PET/CT in the planning of radiotherapy for early-stage Hodgkin lymphoma. Eur J Haematol 2007;78(3):206–12.
6. Terezakis SA, Hunt MA, Kowalski A, et al. (18)F] FDG-positron emission tomography coregistration with computed tomography scans for radiation

treatment planning of lymphoma and hematologic malignancies. Int J Radiat Oncol Biol Phys 2010. [Epub ahead of print].

7. Lee YK, Cook G, Flower MA, et al. Addition of 18F-FDG-PET scans to radiotherapy planning of thoracic lymphoma. Radiother Oncol 2004;73(3):277–83.

8. Ling CC, Humm J, Larson S, et al. Towards multidimensional radiotherapy (MD-CRT): biological imaging and biological conformality. Int J Radiat Oncol Biol Phys 2000;47(3):551–60.

9. Yahalom J, Mauch P. The involved field is back: issues in delineating the radiation field in Hodgkin's disease. Ann Oncol 2002;13(Suppl 1):79–83.

10. Campbell BA, Voss N, Pickles T, et al. Involved-nodal radiation therapy as a component of combination therapy for limited-stage Hodgkin's lymphoma: a question of field size. J Clin Oncol 2008;26(32): 5170–4.

11. Campbell BA, Voss N, Woods R, et al. Long-term outcomes for patients with limited stage follicular lymphoma: involved regional radiotherapy versus involved node radiotherapy. Cancer 2010;116(16): 3797–806.

12. Jerusalem G, Beguin Y, Najjar F, et al. Positron emission tomography (PET) with 18F-fluorodeoxyglucose (18F-FDG) for the staging of low-grade non-Hodgkin's lymphoma (NHL). Ann Oncol 2001;12(6): 825–30.

13. Jerusalem G, Beguin Y, Fassotte MF, et al. Whole-body positron emission tomography using 18F-fluorodeoxyglucose compared to standard procedures for staging patients with Hodgkin's disease. Haematologica 2001;86(3):266–73.

14. Sasaki M, Kuwabara Y, Koga H, et al. Clinical impact of whole body FDG-PET on the staging and therapeutic decision making for malignant lymphoma. Ann Nucl Med 2002;16(5):337–45.

15. Schoder H, Meta J, Yap C, et al. Effect of whole-body (18)F-FDG PET imaging on clinical staging and management of patients with malignant lymphoma. J Nucl Med 2001;42(8):1139–43.

16. Schiepers C, Filmont JE, Czernin J. PET for staging of Hodgkin's disease and non-Hodgkin's lymphoma. Eur J Nucl Med Mol Imaging 2003;30(Suppl 1): S82–8.

17. Weihrauch MR, Re D, Bischoff S, et al. Whole-body positron emission tomography using 18F-fluorodeoxyglucose for initial staging of patients with Hodgkin's disease. Ann Hematol 2002;81(1):20–5.

18. Wirth A, Seymour JF, Hicks RJ, et al. Fluorine-18 fluorodeoxyglucose positron emission tomography, gallium-67 scintigraphy, and conventional staging for Hodgkin's disease and non-Hodgkin's lymphoma. Am J Med 2002;112(4):262–8.

19. Stumpe KD, Urbinelli M, Steinert HC, et al. Whole-body positron emission tomography using fluorodeoxyglucose for staging of lymphoma: effectiveness and comparison with computed tomography. Eur J Nucl Med 1998;25(7):721–8.

20. Hutchings M, Loft A, Hansen M, et al. Different histopathological subtypes of Hodgkin lymphoma show significantly different levels of FDG uptake. Hematol Oncol 2006;24(3):146–50.

21. Newman JS, Francis IR, Kaminski MS, et al. Imaging of lymphoma with PET with 2-[F-18]-fluoro-2-deoxy-D-glucose: correlation with CT. Radiology 1994; 190(1):111–6.

22. Okada J, Yoshikawa K, Itami M, et al. Positron emission tomography using fluorine-18-fluorodeoxyglucose in malignant lymphoma: a comparison with proliferative activity. J Nucl Med 1992;33(3):325–9.

23. Okada J, Yoshikawa K, Imazeki K, et al. The use of FDG-PET in the detection and management of malignant lymphoma: correlation of uptake with prognosis. J Nucl Med 1991;32(4):686–91.

24. Hoffmann M, Kletter K, Becherer A, et al. 18F-fluorodeoxyglucose positron emission tomography (18F-FDG-PET) for staging and follow-up of marginal zone B-cell lymphoma. Oncology 2003;64(4):336–40.

25. Najjar F, Hustinx R, Jerusalem G, et al. Positron emission tomography (PET) for staging low-grade non-Hodgkin's lymphomas (NHL). Cancer Biother Radiopharm 2001;16(4):297–304.

26. Schoder H, Noy A, Gonen M, et al. Intensity of 18fluorodeoxyglucose uptake in positron emission tomography distinguishes between indolent and aggressive non-Hodgkin's lymphoma. J Clin Oncol 2005;23(21):4643–51.

27. Scarfone C, Lavely WC, Cmelak AJ, et al. Prospective feasibility trial of radiotherapy target definition for head and neck cancer using 3-dimensional PET and CT imaging. J Nucl Med 2004;45(4): 543–52.

28. Nishioka T, Shiga T, Shirato H, et al. Image fusion between 18FDG-PET and MRI/CT for radiotherapy planning of oropharyngeal and nasopharyngeal carcinomas. Int J Radiat Oncol Biol Phys 2002; 53(4):1051–7.

29. Schwartz DL, Ford EC, Rajendran J, et al. FDG-PET/CT-guided intensity modulated head and neck radiotherapy: a pilot investigation. Head Neck 2005;27(6):478–87.

30. Kiffer JD, Berlangieri SU, Scott AM, et al. The contribution of 18F-fluoro-2-deoxy-glucose positron emission tomographic imaging to radiotherapy planning in lung cancer. Lung Cancer 1998;19(3):167–77.

31. Nestle U, Walter K, Schmidt S, et al. 18F-deoxyglucose positron emission tomography (FDG-PET) for the planning of radiotherapy in lung cancer: high impact in patients with atelectasis. Int J Radiat Oncol Biol Phys 1999;44(3):593–7.

32. Vanuytsel LJ, Vansteenkiste JF, Stroobants SG, et al. The impact of (18)F-fluoro-2-deoxy-D-glucose positron emission tomography (FDG-PET) lymph node

staging on the radiation treatment volumes in patients with non-small cell lung cancer. Radiother Oncol 2000;55(3):317–24.

33. Giraud P, Grahek D, Montravers F, et al. CT and (18) F-deoxyglucose (FDG) image fusion for optimization of conformal radiotherapy of lung cancers. Int J Radiat Oncol Biol Phys 2001;49(5):1249–57.

34. Caldwell CB, Mah K, Ung YC, et al. Observer variation in contouring gross tumor volume in patients with poorly defined non-small-cell lung tumors on CT: the impact of 18FDG-hybrid PET fusion. Int J Radiat Oncol Biol Phys 2001;51(4):923–31.

35. MacManus MP, Hicks RJ, Ball DL, et al. Imaging with F-18 FDG PET is superior to tl-201 SPECT in the staging of non-small cell lung cancer for radical radiation therapy. Australas Radiol 2001;45(4):483–90.

36. Mah K, Caldwell CB, Ung YC, et al. The impact of (18)FDG-PET on target and critical organs in CT-based treatment planning of patients with poorly defined non-small-cell lung carcinoma: a prospective study. Int J Radiat Oncol Biol Phys 2002;52(2): 339–50.

37. Erdi YE, Rosenzweig K, Erdi AK, et al. Radiotherapy treatment planning for patients with non-small cell lung cancer using positron emission tomography (PET). Radiother Oncol 2002;62(1):51–60.

38. Bradley J, Thorstad WL, Mutic S, et al. Impact of FDG-PET on radiation therapy volume delineation in non-small-cell lung cancer. Int J Radiat Oncol Biol Phys 2004;59(1):78–86.

39. Ciernik IF, Dizendorf E, Baumert BG, et al. Radiation treatment planning with an integrated positron emission and computer tomography (PET/CT): a feasibility study. Int J Radiat Oncol Biol Phys 2003; 57(3):853–63.

40. Rahn AN, Baum RP, Adamietz IA, et al. Value of 18F fluorodeoxyglucose positron emission tomography in radiotherapy planning of head-neck tumors. Strahlenther Onkol 1998;174(7):358–64.

41. Brianzoni E, Rossi G, Ancidei S, et al. Radiotherapy planning: PET/CT scanner performances in the definition of gross tumour volume and clinical target volume. Eur J Nucl Med Mol Imaging 2005;32(12): 1392–9.

42. Girinsky T, Ghalibafian M. Radiotherapy of Hodgkin lymphoma: indications, new fields, and techniques. Semin Radiat Oncol 2007;17(3):206–22.

43. Picardi M, De Renzo A, Pane F, et al. Randomized comparison of consolidation radiation versus observation in bulky Hodgkin's lymphoma with post-chemotherapy negative positron emission tomography scans. Leuk lymphoma 2007;48(9):1721–7.

44. Girinsky T, Specht L, Ghalibafian M, et al. The conundrum of Hodgkin lymphoma nodes: to be or not to be included in the involved node radiation fields. the EORTC-GELA lymphoma group guidelines. Radiother Oncol 2008;88(2):202–10.

45. Pommier P, Touboul E, Chabaud S, et al. Impact of (18)F-FDG PET on treatment strategy and 3D radiotherapy planning in non-small cell lung cancer: a prospective multicenter study. AJR Am J Roentgenol 2010;195(2):350–5.

46. Beyer T, Townsend DW, Brun T, et al. A combined PET/CT scanner for clinical oncology. J Nucl Med 2000;41(8):1369–79.

47. Cohade C, Osman M, Marshall LN, et al. PET-CT: accuracy of PET and CT spatial registration of lung lesions. Eur J Nucl Med Mol Imaging 2003;30(5):721–6.

48. Cohade C, Wahl RL. Applications of positron emission tomography/computed tomography image fusion in clinical positron emission tomography-clinical use, interpretation methods, diagnostic improvements. Semin Nucl Med 2003;33(3):228–37.

49. Fox JL, Rengan R, O'Meara W, et al. Does registration of PET and planning CT images decrease interobserver and intraobserver variation in delineating tumor volumes for non-small-cell lung cancer? Int J Radiat Oncol Biol Phys 2005;62(1):70–5.

50. Heron DE, Andrade RS, Flickinger J, et al. Hybrid PET-CT simulation for radiation treatment planning in head-and-neck cancers: a brief technical report. Int J Radiat Oncol Biol Phys 2004;60(5):1419–24.

51. Riegel AC, Berson AM, Destian S, et al. Variability of gross tumor volume delineation in head-and-neck cancer using CT and PET/CT fusion. Int J Radiat Oncol Biol Phys 2006;65(3):726–32.

52. Breen SL, Publicover J, De Silva S, et al. Intraobserver and interobserver variability in GTV delineation on FDG-PET-CT images of head and neck cancers. Int J Radiat Oncol Biol Phys 2007;68(3):763–70.

53. van Baardwijk A, Bosmans G, Boersma L, et al. PET-CT-based auto-contouring in non-small-cell lung cancer correlates with pathology and reduces interobserver variability in the delineation of the primary tumor and involved nodal volumes. Int J Radiat Oncol Biol Phys 2007;68(3):771–8.

54. Ford EC, Kinahan PE, Hanlon L, et al. Tumor delineation using PET in head and neck cancers: threshold contouring and lesion volumes. Med Phys 2006; 33(11):4280–8.

55. Nestle U, Kremp S, Schaefer-Schuler A, et al. Comparison of different methods for delineation of 18F-FDG PET-positive tissue for target volume definition in radiotherapy of patients with non-small cell lung cancer. J Nucl Med 2005;46(8):1342–8.

56. Daisne JF, Sibomana M, Bol A, et al. Tri-dimensional automatic segmentation of PET volumes based on measured source-to-background ratios: influence of reconstruction algorithms. Radiother Oncol 2003;69(3):247–50.

57. Erdi YE, Mawlawi O, Larson SM, et al. Segmentation of lung lesion volume by adaptive positron emission tomography image thresholding. Cancer 1997; 80(12 Suppl):2505–9.

58. Nehmeh SA, Erdi YE, Ling CC, et al. Effect of respiratory gating on quantifying PET images of lung cancer. J Nucl Med 2002;43(7):876–81.

59. Nehmeh SA, Erdi YE, Ling CC, et al. Effect of respiratory gating on reducing lung motion artifacts in PET imaging of lung cancer. Med Phys 2002;29(3): 366–71.

60. Nehmeh SA, Erdi YE, Pan T, et al. Four-dimensional (4D) PET/CT imaging of the thorax. Med Phys 2004; 31(12):3179–86.

61. Nestle U, Kremp S, Grosu AL. Practical integration of [18F]-FDG-PET and PET-CT in the planning of radiotherapy for non-small cell lung cancer (NSCLC): the technical basis, ICRU-target volumes, problems, perspectives. Radiother Oncol 2006; 81(2):209–25.

62. Ford EC, Mageras GS, Yorke E, et al. Respiration-correlated spiral CT: a method of measuring respiratory-induced anatomic motion for radiation treatment planning. Med Phys 2003;30(1):88–97.

63. Vedam SS, Keall PJ, Kini VR, et al. Acquiring a four-dimensional computed tomography dataset using an external respiratory signal. Phys Med Biol 2003; 48(1):45–62.

The Role of PET in the Evaluation, Treatment, and Ongoing Management of Lung Cancer

Kevin Stephans, MD[a,c,]*, Anton Khouri, MD[a,b],
Mitchell Machtay, MD[a,b]

KEYWORDS

- PET • Radiation • Lung cancer • Staging
- Response assessment

PET has gained a major role in the evaluation and treatment of lung cancer over the past two decades. Over that time span PET and treatment techniques have both evolved substantially. While technical changes in PET and PET/computed tomography (CT) have improved accuracy and reliability, the evolution toward increasingly targeted and intensive treatment has increased the reliance upon imaging for radiation treatment. This article seeks to review the current role of PET in the evaluation and treatment of lung cancer with radiation.

DIAGNOSIS

The PET scan has attained a central role in both the evaluation of new pulmonary lesions and the staging of lung cancer. A meta-analysis of 40 prospective studies suggested a sensitivity of 96.8% and specificity of 77.8%[1] for PET in the evaluation of a new lung nodule. This finding makes PET an excellent frontline study, even prior to pathologic diagnosis of lung cancer. PET is extremely useful in guiding the need for biopsy, given that PET-negative lesions are rarely malignant and therefore can typically be followed clinically. Most PET false-negative lung cancers are bronchoalveolar carcinomas. These lesions have unique CT characteristics and are typically low grade with a slow-growth pattern demonstrating progression over only long intervals, therefore the urgency of diagnosis may be less. As the specificity of PET is only 77.8%,[1] biopsy confirmation of malignancy remains vital. Biopsy offers confirmation of malignancy justifying treatment, as well as histology, which is critical. For example, small cell lung cancer (SCLC) and non–small cell lung cancer (NSCLC) may be treated very differently despite otherwise identical presentation.

Combining PET with CT allows the potential for integrated imaging, which should improve sensitivity by eliminating from consideration areas of increased standardized uptake value (SUV) with no associated CT changes. The specificity of PET/CT might be greater than the 77.8% reported for PET alone in the aforementioned meta-analysis, though comparative data at this point are limited. Some investigators have even suggested that combining CT and PET features may even give some insight into tumor histology[2]; this

This work was done independently of any grant or research funding.
a Department of Radiation Oncology, Cleveland Clinic, 9500 Euclid Avenue, T28, Cleveland, OH 44195, USA
b Department of Radiation Oncology, University Hospitals/Case Western Reserve University, 11100 Euclid Avenue, Cleveland, OH 44106, USA
c Case Comprehensive Cancer Center, Wearn 152, 11100 Euclid Avenue, Cleveland, OH, USA
* Corresponding author. Department of Radiation Oncology, Cleveland Clinic, 9500 Euclid Avenue, T28, Cleveland, OH 44195.
E-mail address: stephak@ccf.org

PET Clin 6 (2011) 177–184
doi:10.1016/j.cpet.2011.02.010
1556-8598/11/$ – see front matter © 2011 Elsevier Inc. All rights reserved.

may take on further interest with the future availability of additional PET tracers.

An important exception to the requirement for tissue diagnosis comes in medically inoperable patients with highly suspected NSCLC. Biopsy may be high risk in patients with extremely poor lung function or in those with history of contralateral pneumonectomy, and otherwise unreliable in patients with small but PET-positive lesions located in areas where access is technically challenging. Such patients are typically treated based on radiographic criteria, which may vary by institution. To consider empiric treatment, a lesion is required to be both increasing in size on serial CT over a 6-week to 3-month interval, and positive on PET with an SUV of greater than 3.0. The numbers of patients treated in this manner are small and the population is heterogeneous, making reliable analysis of these criteria difficult. However, the fact that the rate of future distant metastasis is comparable in a series of stage I patients treated with histologic versus radiographic characteristics suggests these criteria are reasonable.[3]

STAGING

Once a biopsy diagnosis is reached, PET/CT is the gold standard for noninvasive staging. PET offers substantial improvements in both mediastinal and distant staging over CT criteria alone, and is the standard of care for all patients with newly diagnosed NSCLC.

Mediastinal Staging

According to a recent meta-analysis the addition of PET to standard CT increases the sensitivity for the detection of mediastinal nodal involvement from 61% to 85%, while specificity is improved from 79% to 90%.[4] Of interest, when CT demonstrated enlarged mediastinal lymph nodes PET was more sensitive (100%), but less specific than at baseline (78%). Conversely, when CT showed no nodal enlargement, sensitivity was near baseline at 82% and specificity 93%. This finding has important treatment planning implications: enlarged but PET-negative nodes therefore are unlikely to contain disease (as PET was 100% sensitive in this series), whereas small but PET-positive nodes are very likely to be malignant. Given the association of target size and PET SUV measurement, both of these conclusions are logical, and have important implications for both staging and treatment planning.

Even after PET, patients who are surgical candidates frequently proceed to additional staging by mediastinoscopy prior to the final selection of treatment modality. The ACOSOG Z0050 trial[5]

investigated the correlation of CT, PET, and mediastinoscopy in 303 potentially resectable patients with NSCLC. PET detected microscopic N2 nodal disease in 58% of patients. However, as sensitivity was only 61% and negative predictive value 87%, the ability of PET to detect microscopic N2 disease appears to be modest. In addition, a Cleveland Clinic review[6] of 87 patients with pathologic stage IIIA NSCLC by mediastinoscopy reported that 38% of pN2+ patients had no previous abnormal PET findings in the mediastinum. Other reports suggest higher accuracy of PET, including a recent Korean report[7] of 750 NSCLC patients who were mediastinal node negative by CT and PET criteria and who underwent mediastinoscopy. Only 6.8% of these patients were found to have N2 disease on mediastinoscopy, though an additional 8.5% were later found to have N2 disease on final surgical dissection after completion of neoadjuvant therapy. A similar Japanese study[8] suggested an 11% (24 out of 224) incidence of mediastinoscopy-detected microscopic N2 disease present in NSCLC patients who were node negative by PET. Of note, most metastases were small, with two-thirds being less than 4 mm. Multivariate analysis identified adenocarcinoma, tumors located in upper or middle lobe, tumor size larger than 3 cm, and maximum SUV of primary tumor greater than 4.0 g/mL as significant risk factors for microscopic nodal metastasis. An Irish review by Al-Sarraf and colleagues[9] demonstrated a 16% incidence of microscopic N2 disease in PET-negative patients, and identified central tumors, right upper lobe tumors, and PET-positive uptake in hilar (N1) nodes as significant risk factors for undetected microscopic N2 disease. Based on the aforementioned studies the incidence of PET false-negative mediastinal nodes ranges substantially, from 10% to as much as 40%. For this reason mediastinoscopy remains clinically indicated for most patients undergoing surgical resection. Conversely, for patients with locally advanced NSCLC undergoing chemoradiation (as well as medically inoperable stage I NSCLC) mediastinoscopy, an invasive procedure that would delay the start of radiotherapy is not typically performed. The standard staging system for these patients is based on PET. Additional mediastinal staging tools such as endobronchial ultrasound sampling, magnetic resonance (MR) imaging, or MR spectroscopy are currently under investigation as a supplement to PET in these patients.

Despite some limitations in the detection of microscopic disease, PET remains an important supplement to mediastinoscopy. Limitations to mediastinoscopy include variation in the number of nodes sampled by individual surgeons as well as access only to a limited number of mediastinal nodal stations. This is illustrated in a Danish randomized trial[10] of 189 patients to mediastinoscopy with or without preceding PET/CT. The accuracy of nodal staging was improved from 85% to 95% with the addition of PET/CT.

For locally advanced NSCLC patients treated with chemoradiation, as well as stage I medically inoperable NSCLC, mediastinoscopy has not been part of the standard staging with target volumes primarily based on CT, PET, and clinical judgment. The accuracy of staging in this population has been less well studied, with no large cooperative group trials, and is inherently more challenging because of the absence of pathologic confirmation accompanying resection in surgical series. Data assessing the accuracy of staging for nonsurgical patients is therefore based primarily on outcomes, that is, patterns of failure. The overall limited prognosis of many of these patients, due to comorbidities in the medically inoperable stage I population, and progressive disease in the locally advanced chemoradiation population, makes accurate assessment of staging difficult in these settings. Preradiation PET staging alone appears to be justified in stage I NSCLC because isolated nodal failure is less than 5% despite treatment to the primary site alone.[3,11,12] In the locally advanced population, precise staging of the mediastinum has been historically less important because of the widespread use of comprehensive elective nodal radiation. However, mediastinal staging is becoming a topic of greater interest, with modernly tailored fields and selective dose escalation. This trend is discussed in greater detail in the section on treatment planning. The difference between PET and mediastinoscopy staging is important to consider when comparing outcomes of surgical and nonoperative series.

Distant Staging

In addition to improvements in mediastinal nodal staging, PET has substantial impact on treatment choices by improving systemic staging. In the ACOSOG Z0050 trial,[5] 6.3% of patients were found to have extracranial distant metastasis not seen on previous CT staging at the time of PET scan. A meta-analysis of more than 1000 patients[13] suggested a sensitivity of 94% and specificity of 97% in the detection of distant metastasis. Overall there was a 12% rate of detection of distant metastasis, and a change in the therapeutic plan for 18% of patients (in some cases CT-diagnosed metastasis were ruled out)

through the use of PET rather than conventional imaging. PET is excellent at detecting metastasis in otherwise normal-appearing soft tissue (liver, adrenals, omentum, and upper abdominal nodes) as well as in the evaluation of otherwise benign enlargements such as adrenal adenomas and bone islands. The detection of metastasis also increases with increasing stage. MacManus and colleagues[14] found a 7.5% incidence of metastasis in stage I NSCLC, increasing to 18% in stage II and 24% in stage III. As PET is poor at detecting brain metastasis because of high background metabolism, dedicated brain imaging (contrast-enhanced CT or MR imaging) is recommended as a supplement to PET by National Comprehensive Cancer Center guidelines for asymptomatic stage II and higher NSCLC, and is optional for patients with asymptomatic stage I disease (recommended for all patients with central nervous system symptoms). PET is also more accurate than bone scan in evaluation for bone metastasis.[15,16] The only setting where bone scan may be preferred (in combination with serum alkaline phosphatase) is in previously established stage IV disease where PET is not otherwise needed and bone scan may be more cost effective. The same seems to be true for SCLC, where PET appears to be equally accurate as CT plus bone scan and bone marrow analysis, though with more limited data.[17,18]

In summary, PET is recommended for the staging of all patients with a new diagnosis of lung cancer, and has been shown to be cost effective because of its ability to more appropriately select therapeutic choices,[19] which is particularly true in the age of dose-escalated radiotherapy with elimination of elective nodal radiation. This aspect will increase the importance of the staging PET scan, discussed in greater detail below. For patients under evaluation for surgical therapy, mediastinoscopy should supplement PET findings prior to thoracotomy, as microscopic nodal metastasis may be missed by PET in 10% to 40% of cases.

PROGNOSIS

In a systematic review[20] of 13 studies comprising 1474 patients with NSCLC, increasing maximum PET SUV was found to be prognostic as a continuous variable for lower overall survival, though no clear cutoff was identified. This result has been confirmed individually in patients undergoing surgical resection for a range of NSCLCs,[21,22] stage I NSCLC,[23] and chemoradiation for locally advanced NSCLC.[24,25] Of note, the only two studies looking at stereotactic radiation for stage I NSCLC did not find a correlation between maximum pretreatment SUV and local control, distant failure, or overall survival.[26,27] A third study including a large number of stage I NSCLC patients was also inconclusive.[28] The critical unanswered question is whether the mechanism for the relationship of maximal pretreatment PET SUV to affect overall survival is through the inability to control local disease, or rather a higher potential for distant metastasis (or perhaps both). Insight into this would allow for appropriate escalation of therapy, with either additional local therapy or the addition of systemic therapies in appropriately selected patients.

One major limiting confounding factor in answering this question is that because of respiratory motion and other measurement factors, larger tumors will have higher maximum SUV values than similarly active smaller tumors. Tumor size is a known risk factor for both nodal and distant metastasis, and this association between size and SUV may not always be controlled for adequately. For example, in the analysis by Ikushima and colleagues[24] from M.D. Anderson, PET SUV strongly predicted for local control, distant metastasis, and overall survival in a series of 149 patients with locally advanced NSCLC treated with chemoradiation. When tumor size alone was corrected, this association weakened substantially. On multivariate analysis of patients receiving integrated PET/CT, SUV was not significant for any outcome measure.

The lack of correlation of pretreatment PET SUV to outcomes after stereotactic radiation[26–28] is also of interest given its frequent correlation for other treatment modalities; this may simply be due to limited numbers of patients and follow-up in this series. Other potential explanations include the possibility that the extremely dose-escalated treatment overcomes radioresistance. In addition, perhaps the inclusion of low-grade, poorly margined tumors (which may be more challenging to target), particularly in series including patients without biopsy confirmation, introduces the possibility of bimodal distribution of SUV-related outcomes.

Overall it is well established that, in general, tumors with high pretreatment maximum SUV values have inferior prognosis; however, the mechanisms for this are not well established, and there may be differences among disease stages and treatment modalities.

TREATMENT PLANNING

PET imaging has significant implications for treatment volumes, particularly in the setting of locally advanced NSCLC. The impact of improved disease targeting should continue to increase in the newer era of dose-escalated, image-guided radiation to smaller, more precise treatment fields, as this will emphasize the importance of accuracy in field design.

For medically inoperable stage I NSCLC, PET will rarely change treatment fields, outside of the impact on initial staging, as most lesions are well defined given the clear boundary between an isolated pulmonary nodule and surrounding air. Aside from occasional demonstration of clear invasion into the mediastinum, the boundary between tumor and either mediastinum or chest wall is typically more clearly seen on CT or MR imaging. The primary role of PET in delineation of target volumes for stage I NSCLC is in the differentiation of tumor from occasional downstream atelectasis, particularly with larger lesions.

Medically inoperable stage II NSCLC is a relatively uncommon and poorly defined entity. As such, a standard of care does not truly exist and the concept of elective nodal radiation is poorly defined in this context. The primary lesion and ipsilateral hilar nodal regions clearly will be targeted. The use of at least some elective mediastinal nodal radiation is relatively common, given the association of PET-positive hilar nodes to mediastinal micrometastasis. Other previously identified risk factors are tumor size larger than 3 cm, upper or middle lobe tumors, central tumors, primary tumor SUV greater than 4, and adenocarcinoma histology.[8,9] The final decision on field size and mediastinal radiation in these patients is frequently a compromise, weighing the risk factors for mediastinal disease against the patient's overall performance as well as medical comorbidities that prohibited surgery in the first place. Consideration should be given to mediastinoscopy or endobronchial ultrasound sampling in appropriate patients.

In stage III NSCLC, evidence for improved overall survival with dose escalation is mounting. An analysis of data from 7 randomized Radiation Therapy Oncology Group (RTOG) trials demonstrated total radiation dose to be strongly correlated with both local control and overall survival.[29] Each 1-Gy increase in biological equivalent dose was associated with a 4% relative improvement in survival and 3% improvement in local control. Furthermore, a randomized Chinese trial of standard dose radiation with elective nodal coverage versus escalated radiation dose to involved disease alone demonstrated an improvement in 2-year overall survival from 26% to 39% in favor of escalated dose to the involved target volume only.[30] At the same time, toxicity-related breaks in treatment have been shown to have a deleterious effect on survival.[31] As clinical recurrence in areas of omitted elective nodal radiation has been documented to be rare,[30,32–34] there is a strong movement to dose-escalated radiation to involved nodes only, with consideration of elective coverage only to the highest risk mediastinal nodes, to maximize dose while minimizing toxicity. PET is thus a critical tool in identification of the true involved target volume, and has been demonstrated to affect treatment volumes in many stage III patients, changing the electively targeted volume from CT alone along with the corresponding volume of normal lung and esophagus irradiated in the majority of patients.[32–35] RTOG 0515,[32] a recent prospective multicenter cooperative group phase 2 trial, demonstrated a 10% reduction in treatment volumes when adding PET information to CT contours with a corresponding trend to decrease in median lung dose, without significant change in the number of involved nodes or median esophageal dose. Only one patient (2%) had developed an out-of-field elective nodal failure with 12.9-month median follow-up.

PET-guided selective nodal radiation with consideration of escalation of radiation dose is the current standard of care for locally advanced NSCLC based on the aforementioned results.

ADAPTIVE TREATMENT

The concept of adaptive replanning during treatment to adjust for changes in tumor size is most common in head and neck cancer. This concept has gained popularity for this site for two reasons: the observed rapid treatment response of some large neck lymph nodes involved with squamous cell carcinoma; and the resultant change in dosimetry to both normal structures and tumor, due to treatment to a small area of the body with changing surface dimensions and close association of critical tissue. The importance of this concept may be slightly less in lung cancer because of the far lesser extent of changes in surface anatomy during therapy. Nevertheless, with local control rates not much more than 50% even with dose-escalated therapy, there may be room for further escalation and volume reduction. Two studies[36,37] of volume changes with mid-treatment PET scan after 5 to 6 weeks of radiation, with the goal of reduced volume high-dose boost, have demonstrated modest reductions in full-dose radiation target volume by 20% to 44%, though the expected benefit in normal tissue complications averaged only 2%. This is a novel and interesting concept, which at this point remains experimental and requires further study.

RESPONSE ASSESSMENT

The significance of posttreatment imaging changes in NSCLC can be extremely complicated because of the common presence of postradiation fibrosis, atelectasis, and inflammatory changes during the standard follow-up interval. Furthermore, the modest rate of local control, even with modern dose-escalated radiation, provides rationale for consideration of further intensification of therapy if local failure, or at least poor response, can be identified early. This concept has led to interest in the role of PET in response assessment. A prospective Australian study by MacManus and colleagues[38] suggested a much more powerful correlation of outcome to PET metabolic response versus CT response. At a median of 70 days post treatment 2-year overall survivals of 61%, 34%, 20%, and 18% were noted respectively for patients with a metabolic complete response, versus partial response, stable disease, or progressive disease. Furthermore, metabolic complete response was much more common than CT complete response (47% vs 14%), with poor concordance between PET and CT responses. Inflammatory changes were also noted in normal tissue, and appeared to correlate positively with the degree of metabolic tumor response, suggesting linkage between normal tissue radiosensitivity and tumor response.[39] Rosenzweig and colleagues[40] likewise demonstrated improvement in local control of 83% compared with 23% for patients with 4-month postradiation PET SUV of less than 3.5 versus SUV greater than 3.5. Decreases in maximum SUV during and just after treatment have also been shown to correlate with improved survival for both induction chemotherapy[41] and chemoradiation.[25] A large prospective multi-institutional trial of PET response to chemoradiation (ACRIN 6668/RTOG 0235) has recently been completed, with results pending.[42] These data will help further establish the role of PET in the early posttreatment response assessment, and likely will serve as a springboard for further attempts to improve outcome.

Although the field of stereotactic radiation (SBRT) for NSCLC is relatively new, early data are available regarding PET response to treatment. These data are of increased interest to SBRT given the high incidence of posttreatment inflammatory changes, which can be very intense, prolonged, and easily mistaken for tumor progression. As part of a prospective pilot study,[43] 14 patients treated to 60 Gy in 3 fractions underwent repeat PET at 2, 26, and 52 weeks after SBRT. While maximum SUV values generally decreased over time, the median was higher at 52 weeks than at 26 weeks. Six patients with maximum SUV remaining above 3.5 had no evidence of local progression with further follow-up (the only patient with a persistently rising SUV had repeat biopsy negative for disease, but died shortly thereafter of infection, limiting further follow-up data). A similar study from Georgetown[44] evaluating 20 patients demonstrated some mild individual elevations in maximum SUV, though the average decreased from 6.2 to 2.3. At 18 to 24 months, however, controlled tumors showed a narrow range of SUVs (1.5 to 2.8), whereas a single confirmed local failure exhibited an SUV of 8.4. Additional data will be derived from RTOG 0618, which is a prospective multi-institutional trial of SBRT in medically operable patients and includes posttreatment PET evaluation for identification of patients for surgical salvage.[45] Further investigation is needed, although early results suggest occasional early reactive increase in SUV but long-term declines in controlled patients. Thus any patient with a persistently elevated or increasing SUV should be evaluated and given the potential for salvage therapy. Elevated SUV alone, however, should not be automatically assumed to represent recurrence/progression, and repeat biopsy is strongly recommended. Assessment of post-SBRT PET response will gain increasing importance as a trigger for biopsy and/or surgical salvage with increasing use of SBRT in medically operable early-stage NSCLC.

NOVEL DIRECTIONS

^{18}F-Fluoro-D-deoxyglucose PET is well established. However, a host of other tracers that are analogues to thymidine, methionine, choline, annexin V, as well as proliferative and hypoxic markers, plus a variety of other cellular activity markers are under further investigation. These agents may help clarify the biological blueprint of tumors to identify prognosis, give insight into tumor histology, predict toxicity and, more significantly, lead to novel methods of treatment selection and targeted therapies. Along with mapping of tumor DNA and protein, as well as MR spectroscopy, novel PET analogues represent the horizon of individualized tumor therapy, though substantial prospective assessment is required before the clinical impact can be confirmed and realized.

SUMMARY

PET is central to the diagnosis and staging of lung cancer. The transition to dose-escalate radiation with increasingly selective nodal radiation has made the accurate characterization of nodal status critical to successful treatment. Although mediastinoscopy increases the detection of microscopic nodal metastasis to a greater extent than PET alone, treatment failure in omitted elective nodal areas is rare with PET-guided modern chemoradiation. New horizons for PET scanning include the ability to potentially allow for early detection of salvageable poor treatment responses or local recurrence, as well as to improve the molecular blueprint of tumors with novel tracers to assist with treatment selection and delivery of targeted therapy. The role of PET imaging in the management of lung cancer is likely to continue to increase in the future.

REFERENCES

1. Gould MK, Maclean CC, Kuschner WG, et al. Accuracy of positron emission tomography for diagnosis of pulmonary nodules and mass lesions: a meta-analysis. JAMA 2001;285(7):914–24.
2. Sun JS, Park KJ, Sheen SS, et al. Clinical usefulness of the fluorodeoxyglucose (FDG)-PET maximal standardized uptake value (SUV) in combination with CT features for the differentiation of adenocarcinoma with a bronchioloalveolar carcinoma from other subtypes of non-small cell lung cancers. Lung Cancer 2009;66(2):205–10.
3. Stephans KL, Djemil T, Reddy CA, et al. A comparison of two stereotactic body radiation fractionation schedules for medically inoperable stage I non-small cell lung cancer: the Cleveland Clinic experience. J Thorac Oncol 2009;4(8):976–82.
4. Gould MK, Kuschner WG, Rydzak CE, et al. Test performance of positron emission tomography and computed tomography for mediastinal staging in patients with non-small-cell lung cancer: a meta-analysis. Ann Intern Med 2003;139(11):879–92.
5. Reed CE, Harpole DH, Posther KE, et al. Results of the American College of Surgeons Oncology Group Z0050 trial: the utility of positron emission tomography in staging potentially operable non-small cell lung cancer. J Thorac Cardiovasc Surg 2003;126(6):1943–51.
6. Videtic GM, Rice TW, Murthy S, et al. Utility of positron emission tomography compared with mediastinoscopy for delineating involved lymph nodes in stage III lung cancer: insights for radiotherapy planning from a surgical cohort. Int J Radiat Oncol Biol Phys 2008;72(3):702–6.
7. Kim HK, Choi YS, Kim K, et al. Outcomes of mediastinoscopy and surgery with or without neoadjuvant therapy in patients with non-small cell lung cancer who are N2 negative on positron emission tomography and computed tomography. J Thorac Oncol 2011;6(2):336–42.

8. Kanzaki R, Higashiyama M, Fujiwara A, et al. Occult mediastinal lymph node metastasis in NSCLC patients diagnosed as clinical N0-1 by preoperative integrated FDG-PET/CT and CT: risk factors, pattern, and histopathological study. Lung Cancer 2011; 71(3):333–7.

9. Al-Sarraf N, Aziz R, Gately K, et al. Pattern and predictors of occult mediastinal lymph node involvement in non-small cell lung cancer patients with negative mediastinal uptake on positron emission tomography. Eur J Cardiothorac Surg 2008;33(1): 104–9.

10. Fischer BM, Mortensen J, Hansen H, et al. Multimodality approach to mediastinal staging in non-small cell lung cancer. Faults and benefits of PET-CT: a randomised trial. Thorax 2010. [Epub ahead of print].

11. Bradley JD, El Naqa I, Drzymala RE, et al. Stereotactic body radiation therapy for early-stage non-small-cell lung cancer: the pattern of failure is distant. Int J Radiat Oncol Biol Phys 2010;77(4): 1146–50.

12. Timmerman R, Paulus R, Galvin J, et al. Stereotactic body radiation therapy for inoperable early stage lung cancer. JAMA 2010;303(11):1070–6.

13. Hellwig D, Ukena D, Paulsen F, et al. Meta-analysis of the efficacy of positron emission tomography with F-18-fluorodeoxyglucose in lung tumors. Basis for discussion of the German Consensus Conference on PET in Oncology 2000. Pneumologie 2001;55(8):367–77.

14. MacManus MP, Hicks RJ, Matthews JP, et al. High rate of detection of unsuspected distant metastases by PET in apparent stage III non-small-cell lung cancer: implications for radical radiation therapy. Int J Radiat Oncol Biol Phys 2001;50(2): 287–93.

15. Ak I, Sivrikoz MC, Entok E, et al. Discordant findings in patients with non-small-cell lung cancer: absolutely normal bone scans versus disseminated bone metastases on positron-emission tomography/computed tomography. Eur J Cardiothorac Surg 2010;37(4):792–6.

16. Song JW, Oh YM, Shim TS, et al. Efficacy comparison between (18)F-FDG PET/CT and bone scintigraphy in detecting bony metastases of non-small-cell lung cancer. Lung Cancer 2009;65(3): 333–8.

17. Bradley JD, Dehdashti F, Mintun MA, et al. Positron emission tomography in limited-stage small-cell lung cancer: a prospective study. J Clin Oncol 2004;22(16):3248–54.

18. Fischer BM, Mortensen J, Langer SW, et al. A prospective study of PET/CT in initial staging of small-cell lung cancer: comparison with CT, bone scintigraphy and bone marrow analysis. Ann Oncol 2007;18(2):338–45.

19. Schreyogg J, Weller J, Stargardt T, et al. Cost-effectiveness of hybrid PET/CT for staging of non-small cell lung cancer. J Nucl Med 2010;51(11): 1668–75.

20. Paesmans M, Berghmans T, Dusart M, et al. Primary tumor standardized uptake value measured on fluorodeoxyglucose positron emission tomography is of prognostic value for survival in non-small cell lung cancer: update of a systematic review and meta-analysis by the European Lung Cancer Working Party for the International Association for the Study of Lung Cancer Staging Project. J Thorac Oncol 2010;5(5):612–9.

21. Downey RJ, Akhurst T, Gonen M, et al. Preoperative F-18 fluorodeoxyglucose-positron emission tomography maximal standardized uptake value predicts survival after lung cancer resection. J Clin Oncol 2004;22(16):3255–60.

22. Okereke IC, Gangadharan SP, Kent MS, et al. Standard uptake value predicts survival in non-small cell lung cancer. Ann Thorac Surg 2009;88(3):911–5 [discussion: 915–6].

23. Nair VS, Barnett PG, Ananth L, et al. PET scan ^{18}F-fluorodeoxyglucose uptake and prognosis in patients with resected clinical stage IA non-small cell lung cancer. Chest 2010;137(5):1150–6.

24. Ikushima H, Dong L, Erasmus J, et al. Predictive value of ^{18}F-fluorodeoxyglucose uptake by positron emission tomography for non-small cell lung cancer patients treated with radical radiotherapy. J Radiat Res (Tokyo) 2010;51(4):465–71.

25. Zhang HQ, Yu JM, Meng X, et al. Prognostic value of serial [(18)F]fluorodeoxyglucose PET-CT uptake in stage III patients with non-small cell lung cancer treated by concurrent chemoradiotherapy. Eur J Radiol 2011;77(1):92–6.

26. Burdick MJ, Stephans KL, Reddy CA, et al. Maximum standardized uptake value from staging FDG-PET/CT does not predict treatment outcome for early-stage non-small-cell lung cancer treated with stereotactic body radiotherapy. Int J Radiat Oncol Biol Phys 2010;78(4):1033–9.

27. Hoopes DJ, Tann M, Fletcher JW, et al. FDG-PET and stereotactic body radiotherapy (SBRT) for stage I non-small-cell lung cancer. Lung Cancer 2007; 56(2):229–34.

28. Coon D, Gokhale AS, Burton SA, et al. Fractionated stereotactic body radiation therapy in the treatment of primary, recurrent, and metastatic lung tumors: the role of positron emission tomography/computed tomography-based treatment planning. Clin Lung Cancer 2008;9(4):217–21.

29. Machtay M, Bae K, Movsas B, et al. Higher biologically effective dose of radiotherapy is associated with improved outcomes for locally advanced non-small cell lung carcinoma treated with chemoradiation: an analysis of the Radiation Therapy Oncology

Group. Int J Radiat Oncol Biol Phys 2010. [Epub ahead of print].

30. Yuan S, Sun X, Li M, et al. A randomized study of involved-field irradiation versus elective nodal irradiation in combination with concurrent chemotherapy for inoperable stage III nonsmall cell lung cancer. Am J Clin Oncol 2007;30(3):239–44.

31. Machtay M, Hsu C, Komaki R, et al. Effect of overall treatment time on outcomes after concurrent chemoradiation for locally advanced non-small-cell lung carcinoma: analysis of the Radiation Therapy Oncology Group (RTOG) experience. Int J Radiat Oncol Biol Phys 2005;63(3):667–71.

32. Bradley J, Bae K, Choi N, et al. A phase II comparative study of gross tumor volume definition with or without PET/CT fusion in dosimetric planning for non-small-cell lung cancer (NSCLC): primary analysis of Radiation Therapy Oncology Group (RTOG) 0515. Int J Radiat Oncol Biol Phys 2010. [Epub ahead of print].

33. Fernandes AT, Shen J, Finlay J, et al. Elective nodal irradiation (ENI) vs. involved field radiotherapy (IFRT) for locally advanced non-small cell lung cancer (NSCLC): a comparative analysis of toxicities and clinical outcomes. Radiother Oncol 2010;95(2): 178–84.

34. Sulman EP, Komaki R, Klopp AH, et al. Exclusion of elective nodal irradiation is associated with minimal elective nodal failure in non-small cell lung cancer. Radiat Oncol 2009;4:5.

35. Bradley J, Thorstad WL, Mutic S, et al. Impact of FDG-PET on radiation therapy volume delineation in non-small-cell lung cancer. Int J Radiat Oncol Biol Phys 2004;59(1):78–86.

36. Feng M, Kong FM, Gross M, et al. Using fluorodeoxyglucose positron emission tomography to assess tumor volume during radiotherapy for non-small-cell lung cancer and its potential impact on adaptive dose escalation and normal tissue sparing. Int J Radiat Oncol Biol Phys 2009;73(4):1228–34.

37. Gillham C, Zips D, Ponisch F, et al. Additional PET/CT in week 5-6 of radiotherapy for patients with stage III non-small cell lung cancer as a means of dose escalation planning? Radiother Oncol 2008; 88(3):335–41.

38. MacManus MP, Hicks RJ, Matthews JP, et al. Positron emission tomography is superior to computed tomography scanning for response-assessment after radical radiotherapy or chemoradiotherapy in patients with non-small-cell lung cancer. J Clin Oncol 2003;21(7):1285–92.

39. Hicks RJ, MacManus MP, Matthews JP, et al. Early FDG-PET imaging after radical radiotherapy for non-small-cell lung cancer: inflammatory changes in normal tissues correlate with tumor response and do not confound therapeutic response evaluation. Int J Radiat Oncol Biol Phys 2004;60(2):412–8.

40. Rosenzweig KE, Fox JL, Giraud P. Response to radiation. Semin Radiat Oncol 2004;14(4):322–5.

41. Eschmann SM, Friedel G, Paulsen F, et al. Repeat ^{18}F-FDG PET for monitoring neoadjuvant chemotherapy in patients with stage III non-small cell lung cancer. Lung Cancer 2007;55(2):165–71.

42. ACRIN 6668/RTOG 0235. Available at: http://www.acrin.org/TabID/155/Default.aspx. Accessed January 31, 2011.

43. Henderson MA, Hoopes DJ, Fletcher JW, et al. A pilot trial of serial ^{18}F-fluorodeoxyglucose positron emission tomography in patients with medically inoperable stage I non-small-cell lung cancer treated with hypofractionated stereotactic body radiotherapy. Int J Radiat Oncol Biol Phys 2010; 76(3):789–95.

44. Vahdat S, Oermann EK, Collins SP, et al. CyberKnife radiosurgery for inoperable stage IA non-small cell lung cancer: ^{18}F-fluorodeoxyglucose positron emission tomography/computed tomography serial tumor response assessment. J Hematol Oncol 2010;3:6.

45. RTOG 0618. Available at: http://www.rtog.org/members/protocols/0618/0618.pdf. Accessed January 31, 2011.

Impact of PET/CT-Based Radiation Therapy Planning in Gastrointestinal Malignancies

Chiaojung Jillian Tsai, MD, PhD, Prajnan Das, MD, MS, MPH*

KEYWORDS

- FDG-PET • PET/CT • Radiation therapy
- Gastrointestinal malignancies

The integration of ^{18}F-flurodeoxyglucose (FDG-PET) with CT images has been widely used in tumor staging and radiation treatment planning of many tumor sites, especially head and neck and non–small cell lung cancers.[1–10] In addition, PET has been increasingly used for treatment monitoring, and findings on PET during cancer treatment can be used to predict treatment outcomes for many cancer sites.[11] Hillner and colleagues[12] demonstrated that physicians often modified their intended chemotherapy or radiation treatment plans when PET was used for treatment monitoring, and the impact of follow-up PET was most significant if it showed worse prognosis compared with the baseline images.

FDG-PET/CT could potentially improve patient management by providing more precise clinical staging and better tumor volume delineation for radiation treatment purposes. For non–small cell lung cancer, the addition of PET/CT in radiation treatment planning has been shown to improve tumor staging and target volume definition.[1–3,6,9] Similar results were also observed in head and neck cancers and other cancer sites.[4,5,7,8,10] For cancers of the gastrointestinal tract, the potential benefit of FDG-PET in radiation therapy management is less studied. This article provides an overview of the available literature concerning the use and impact of PET/CT in radiation treatment planning for cancers of the esophagus/gastroesophageal junction, pancreas, rectum, and anal canal.

CANCER OF THE ESOPHAGUS AND GASTROESOPHAGEAL JUNCTION

The current gold standard for treatment planning is CT-based target volume definition. The relative homogeneity of soft tissue structures surrounding the esophagus makes it difficult, however, to distinguish pathologic features on CT, leading to a potential increase in interobserver variability and a decrease in accuracy. In addition, the cranial and caudal tumor border may be unclear if the esophagus lumen is collapsed and the stomach is not fully expanded.[13] CT also has lower sensitivity and specificity in detecting lymph node metastases compared with FDG-PET.[14–16] Recent advancement of PET/CT technology with fast PET scan time offers an attractive alternative to CT-based planning because PET/CT provides higher accuracy in identifying physiologic and pathologic changes, thereby reducing interobserver variability and increasing accuracy in disease staging.[17–19] Several studies have evaluated the impact of PET/CT on radiation treatment planning,

Department of Radiation Oncology, The University of Texas MD Anderson Cancer Center, 1515 Holcombe Boulevard, Unit 97, Houston, TX 77030, USA
* Corresponding author.
E-mail address: prajdas@mdanderson.org

PET Clin 6 (2011) 185–193
doi:10.1016/j.cpet.2011.02.002
1556-8598/11/$ – see front matter © 2011 Elsevier Inc. All rights reserved.

including the delineation of target volume, observer variability, detection of locoregional lymph node involvement, evaluation of disease staging and metastasis, and radiation dose to nearby structures.[8,9,13,20–30]

Tumor Length/Volume and Geographic Misses

Many studies have investigated the effect of PET/CT on target volumes. In a retrospective study by Schreurs and colleagues[20] of 28 patients with primarily distal esophageal or gastroesophageal junction cancers, PET/CT was found to have the potential to decrease geographic misses. PET/CT affected target volume definition in cranial and/or caudal direction in 61% of the patients, with 11% of the volume from PET/CT-based clinical tumor volume (CTV) located outside the CT-based target volumes. Similarly, Leong and colleagues[13] showed that CT-based gross tumor volume (GTV) excluded FDG-PET–avid disease in 11 of 21 (69%) patients under study, and PET-avid disease was excluded in 31% patients if CT data alone were used, resulting in a geographic miss. In a study of 25 esophageal cancer patients by Hong and colleagues,[25] the use of PET/CT with both semiautomatic and manual contouring techniques also affected target definition. The use of manually defined PET/CT changed the volumes in 21 of 25 (84%) patients; 12 (48%) had minor changes where superior and/or inferior extent of the primary tumor differed by 1 to 2 cm, and 9 patients (36%) had major changes where the difference was greater than 2 cm. A major change was shown in 4 patients (16%) due to a difference in celiac or distant mediastinal lymph node definition. Likewise, Mujis and colleagues[22] demonstrated that PET/CT led to changes in CT-based target volume definition in 12 of 21 patients (57%), 9 of whom had reduction and 3 had increase in tumor volume. The volume defined by PET/CT was inadequately covered by the CT-based treatment plan in 8 patients (36%), and PET-avid GTV was excluded by the CT-based GTV in 13 of 21 patients (61%).[22] Furthermore, Gondi and colleagues[9] found that the addition of PET/CT resulted in smaller GTVs than their CT-based counterparts, with a conformality index of 0.46 (a value of 1 indicates identical PET/CT-based and CT-based GTVs and 0 means no overlap between the 2 volumes). According to Vrieze and colleagues,[30] there seemed to be a 47% discordance (14 of 30 patients) in detecting pathologic lymph nodes between CT/endoscopic ultrasound (EUS) and PET. CT/EUS identified pathologic lymph nodes in 8 patients

that were not detected by PET, and PET showed previously undetected pathologic nodes in 6 patients. Three patients had decreased irradiated volume and 3 had increased volume after the addition of PET.[30] In a separate investigation by Moureau-Zabotto and colleagues,[26] the addition of PET/CT resulted in decreased GTVs in 12 of 34 patients (35%), with a greater than or equal to 25% reduction in 4 patients secondary to decreased tumor lengths. Additionally, the GTV was increased in 7 (21%) patients, and 2 of them had a greater than or equal to 25% increase due to detection of occult disease.[26] Konski and colleagues[29] also reported decreased mean tumor lengths using PET/CT compared with those determined by CT (5.4 cm vs 6.8 cm).

Lymph Node Status/Distant Metastasis

Leong and colleagues[13] showed that the addition of PET/CT information changed the clinical stage in 8 of 21 (38%) patients in a prospective study—4 (19%) patients were upstaged from M0 to M1 due to distant metastasis detected by PET and another 4 (19%) were upstaged from N0 to N1 due to regional lymph node disease previously undetected by CT. This led to a change in treatment from radical chemoradiation to palliative therapy in 5 (24%) patients.

A study conducted by Schreurs and colleagues[24] reported similar results: nodal staging changed in 18 of 61 (30%) patients with esophageal cancer after the PET/CT fusion, and 9 patients had improved certainty in localization of metastatic disease. Furthermore, the disease became upstaged in 1 patient (2%) and downstaged in 3 (5%) patients. Similarly, among the 34 esophageal carcinoma patients referred for concomitant radiotherapy and chemotherapy with curative intent, Moreau-Zabotto and colleagues[26] used PET/CT to identify previously undetected distant metastatic disease in 2 patients (one with hepatic metastases and the other with axillary lymph node metastases), making them ineligible for curative radiation therapy.

Shimizu and colleagues,[21] however, showed the contrary. The investigators analyzed data from 20 esophageal squamous cell carcinoma patients who received CT, EUS, and PET/CT followed by radical surgery and histopathologic examinations of lymph nodes. Out of the 20 patients, subclinical positive lymph node metastasis were detected by CT alone in 8 patients, by CT and EUS in 5 patients, by PET/CT alone in 7 patients, and by PET/CT and EUS in 5 patients. The detection rate of subclinical lymph nodes did not improve after the addition of PET/CT.

Observer Variability

There are mixed results in observer variability when comparing PET/CT with CT in treatment planning. Schreurs and colleagues[20] evaluated interobserver variability in volume definition by comparing CT and PET/CT treatment planning in 28 patients. Tumor volumes were delineated blindly by 3 radiation oncologists using both CT alone and software-based PET/CT fusion. The 3 radiation oncologists were then grouped into 3 two-person pairs, and interobserver concordance indices were computed for each pair. The concordant indices from different pairs of radiation oncologists ranged from 63% to 76% for different target volumes, and there was no significant difference in interobserver variability between CT and PET/CT. In a separate report of 10 patients with gastroesophageal junction cancer by Vesprini and colleagues,[28] GTVs were defined by 6 radiation oncologists independently using CT data first, followed by coregistered PET/CT data. The interobserver and intraobserver variability rates were measured using the standard deviations for tumor length and volume (lymph nodes not included). The median standard deviations for tumor length based on CT alone were significantly greater than those obtained by PET/CT (10 mm vs 8 mm, $P = .02$). The addition of PET/CT also increased volume overlap between observers and there was significantly less intraobserver variability. Overall, the median standard deviations in length and volume as well as the observer agreement index were improved by using PET/CT in treatment planning.

The variability of tumor volume and lengths from different imaging modalities can also be attributed in part to differences in PET/CT uptake threshold values. Yu and colleagues[31] designed a study to evaluate GTV delineation and optimal threshold of tumor length using PET/CT with different uptake value thresholds. For each patient in the study, 5 GTVs were obtained: 1 GTV was defined by CT, 4 GTVs were defined by PET/CT based on different threshold values, and 1 GTV was obtained from surgically resected esophagus specimen. Similarly, 6 measurements of tumor length were obtained for each patient. Using the pathologically derived GTV and tumor length from surgical specimen as the gold standard, the author found that standardized uptake value background SUV of esophagus (SUVbdg) + 20% (SUVmaximum SUV of every slice of the lesion max[slice] − SUVbgd) offered the most optimal

estimate of GTV and length but with an undesirable conformity index (0.52 ± 0.16).

Radiation Doses to Other Organs

There was limited information about the impact of PET/CT on radiation dose to nearby organs. Moreau-Zabotto and colleagues[26] showed that among 34 esophageal cancer patients under study, 12 of them had a reduced percentage of total lung volume receiving greater than 20 Gy (median reduction of 29.4%) after PET/CT image fusion. The percentage of total lung volume receiving greater than 20 Gy was increased in another 12 patients, with a median increase of 25.9%. The maximum spinal doses for CT and PET/CT were comparable, and the percentage of total heart volume receiving greater than 36 Gy increased in 11 patients but decreased in 12 patients.

In summary, combined PET/CT was shown to improve tumor volume delineation and decrease geographic misses when compared with CT alone. In many cases, the addition of PET/CT led to reduction of GTV due to reduction in the longitudinal extent of the disease, and the increase of GTV was secondary to previously undetected lymph node or distant metastasis. The majority of discordance between CT and PET/CT was attributable to differences in tumor delineation in cranial and/or caudal extent of the disease. In some cases, PET/CT also had a significant impact on tumor staging. Interobserver and intraobserver variability remains an important issue, although one study did find improvement when using PET/CT in treatment planning. Overall, the addition of PET/CT does seem to have an impact on radiation treatment planning for esophageal cancer, although its long-term effect on treatment outcome remains unclear.

PANCREATIC CANCER

Patients with locally advanced pancreatic cancer often undergo radiation therapy, and CT-based radiation treatment planning remains the current standard method of choice.[32,33] Compared with FDG-PET, however, CT alone has a low sensitivity and specificity in delineating the primary pancreatic tumor as well as in defining the adjacent lymphatic extension and distant metastasis disease.[34–37] Consequently, it is reasonable to hypothesize that supplementing CT with PET imaging may help better define GTV and planning target volume (PTV), thus reducing geographic misses and improving local disease control.

There are limited data on the impact of PET/CT-based radiation treatment planning on patients with locally advanced pancreatic cancer. Topkan and colleagues[38] have compared CT with PET/CT in GTV delineation in patients with locally advanced, unresectable, pancreatic carcinoma. The investigators found that of the 14 patients in the study, significant GTV changes were seen in 5 patients (35.7%) after using PET/CT for treatment planning. Among all 5 patients, the mean increases in GTV and corresponding PTV were 29.7% (95% CI, 18.2–40.6) and 13.4% (95% CI, 8.6–21.3), respectively. Four of the 5 patients had changes in GTV due to detection of primary tumor beyond the CT-defined tumor limits and 1 patient had additional lymph node metastases detected by PET/CT. For the whole-study population, PET/CT-based treatment planning also led to an increase in both the mean GTVs (104.5 vs 92.5 cm^3) and PTVs (535.2 vs 479.4 cm^3) when compared with CT-based planning. There was no clinically significant difference in the percentage of the PTV dose to adjacent critical organs except for the right kidney, which had a mean of 5.3% increase in radiation exposure with PET/CT based planning.

In addition to 3-D conformal radiation therapy, stereotactic radiation therapy has been used to treat pancreatic tumor plus a defined margin to account for patient motion and misalignment during treatment.[39,40] Stereotactic radiation therapy for pancreatic cancer seems to be associated with higher rates of treatment-related toxicity, however, including duodenal ulcer and perforation.[41,42] So far, no study has evaluated the impact of PET/CT on stereotactic radiation therapy planning for pancreatic cancer treatment. One study looked at the prognostic value of preradiation PET/CT on the outcomes of stereotactic radiation and found that pretreatment PET/CT parameters (maximum standardized uptake value of the tumor) were independent predictors of overall survival after radiation therapy.[43] Although 4-D CT scans and PET were incorporated into the treatment planning process and the fused PET scan was used to guide GTV contouring, no comparison between CT-contoured and PET/CT-contoured tumor characteristics were made. Furthermore, duodenal toxicity remained a significant issue even with PET/CT-based treatment planning.[42]

Taken together, PET/CT-based target volume delineation in patients with locally advanced pancreatic cancer can be theoretically useful. Nevertheless, there have been virtually no data on how PET/CT-based radiation treatment planning might affect target volume definition, geographic misses, and locoregional treatment failures. Although PET/CT-based treatment has been used in stereotactic radiation therapy for pancreatic cancer, the effect of adding PET/CT is unclear. At this point, it is uncertain whether or not PET/CT has any advantage over CT in radiation treatment planning for pancreatic cancer.

RECTAL CANCER

PET/CT has been an established imaging modality for detecting rectal cancer recurrence[44]; however, it has not been widely used as a tool for preoperative staging. A few studies have evaluated the use of FDG-PET for rectal cancer staging and predicting response to preoperative treatment.[45–54] Compared with CT, FDG-PET in general has a relatively high but variable sensitivity and specificity in defining rectal cancer mass and margin, likely attributable to inflammatory reactions around the tumor and differences in standard uptake value thresholds.[49–53] So far, only a few studies have investigated the clinical impact of PET/CT on radiation therapy planning in rectal cancer patients.[8,53–57]

Tumor Volume and Geographic Misses

In a study by Bassi and colleagues,[53] 25 newly diagnosed rectal cancer patients underwent preoperative PET/CT for tumor staging. In addition, GTV and CTV were delineated on both CT and PET/CT, and tumor volumes defined by the two imaging modalities were compared. Overall, the GTV defined by PET/CT was significantly greater than that defined by CT (P<.001), with a mean difference of 25.4% (19.6 ± 29.0 cm^3) of the CT-derived GTV. Similarly, CTV from PET/CT was significantly larger than CTV from CT (P<.001), with a mean difference of 4.1% (29.0 ± 15.2 cm^3) of the CT-based CTV. The changes in tumor volumes were seen at both primary tumor and regional lymph nodes. Likewise, Ciernik and colleagues[8] found that PET/CT led to a 20% increase of PTV secondary to an increase of GTV in 3 of 6 rectal cancer patients undergoing preoperative radiation therapy.

In a retrospective analysis of 36 locally advanced rectal cancer patients by Paskeviciute and colleagues,[54] the investigators showed that the mean GTV from PET/CT was significantly smaller than GTV from CT (62 vs 163 cm^3, P<.05), with a 31% mean volume overlap between the two GTVs. The percentage volume overlap increased with larger GTV from PET/CT, indicating a smaller variation with larger tumor mass. In 16 of 35 patients (46%), traditional PTVs derived from CT would have missed part of the PTV derived from PET/CT, leading to potential geographic misses. This necessitated treatment modifications for these patients. Similar findings were also observed by Anderson and colleagues[57]—PET/CT generated a smaller GTV than that from CT (92 vs 100 cm[3], P<.001), with a 46.7% volume overlap. In 3 of 20 patients (15%), information from PET/CT also resulted in change of PTV. The overlaps of PET/CT and CT-based tumor volume increased significantly with increase in tumor volume.[57]

Another series conducted by Roels and colleagues[58] showed significant discordances between tumor volumes defined by FDG-PET/CT and MR imaging before, during, and after preoperative chemoradiation therapy. FDG-PET tumor volume derived from gradient-based method, however, showed the closest match to pathologic findings—MR imaging demonstrated suspicious residual tumor in 6 of 6 patients with complete pathologic response, whereas FDG-PET exhibited complete metabolic response in 3 of them.[58]

Lymph Node Status/Distant Metastasis

The addition of PET/CT has been shown to affect treatment plans due to changes in tumor staging. Bassi and colleagues[53] found that PET/CT revealed positive nodal disease in the perirectal and presacral regions in 3 of 25 patients (12%) previously staged N0 on CT. In 1 patient with previously diagnosed single hepatic lesion by CT, PET/CT identified multiple liver metastases, thus changing the treatment from curative to palliative intent.[53] Similarly, the study of Paskeviciute and colleagues[54] demonstrated newly identified distant metastasis by PET/CT in 2 of 36 patients. In the same study, overall management and treatment intent was changed from definitive to palliative in 3 of 36 patients (8%): 1 patient had newly diagnosed bone metastases and 2 had detection of multiple liver lesions by PET/CT.[54] Anderson and colleagues[57] also showed that 5 of 20 rectal cancer patients (20%) had a change in overall management, primarily due to identification of previously unrecognized distant diseases. Likewise, Calvo and colleagues[49] and Gerhart and colleagues[51] demonstrated that PET/CT altered tumor staging and therapeutic intent in their studies.

Observer and Tumor Volume Variability

Patel and colleagues[56] evaluated the impact of FDG-PET/CT and ^{18}F-flurodeoxythymidine (FLT)-PET/CT on interobserver variability of target volume definition. In their study, 4 radiation oncologists independently contoured primary and nodal GTVs on CT, FDG-PET/CT, and FLT-PET/CT for a hypothetic boost treatment. A similarity index (with values ranging from 0 to 1—complete

disagreement to complete agreement) was used for each set of volumes to asses interobserver variability. Results from the study showed that both FDG-PET/CT and FLT-PET/CT had significantly higher similarity indices and lower interobserver variability when compared with CT, especially for nodal GTVs. The similarity index was 0.22 for CT-based GTV, 0.70 for GTV from FDG-PET/CT, and 0.70 for GTV from FLT-PET/CT. The findings suggested that PET/CT might offer more uniformity and precision in radiation treatment planning.

Other investigators also evaluated methods of optimizing accuracy in tumor volume definition and reducing variations between CT-derived and PET/CT-derived volumes. For intensity-modulated radiation therapy, Ciernick and colleagues[55] demonstrated that when using a special software tool and a predefined FDG-PET peak threshold value (40% of the signal of interest) to automatically delineate the appropriate tumor volume by FDG signal, a strong correlation between CT-based and PET/CT-derived GTV could be achieved. With adequate extension margins, the automated segmentation of PET signal from rectal cancer could possibly provide relatively accurate definition of PTV for preoperative intensity-modulated radiation therapy.[55]

In conclusion, PET/CT may have a potential impact on preoperative rectal cancer staging and radiation treatment planning. It seems to be capable of reducing geographic misses associated with CT-based planning, and its high sensitivity in detecting locoregional and distant disease involvements might provide valuable information for treatment decision making. In addition, tumor volumes derived from PET/CT have potentially lower interobserver variations when compared with CT-based volume delineation. Typical radiation fields for rectal cancer, however, encompass pelvic nodal regions and not just the primary rectal tumor. Hence, changes in tumor volume delineation may not always have a major impact on the overall radiation field. Further research is needed in elucidating the impact of PET/CT on radiation therapy planning for rectal cancer.

ANAL CANCER

Chemoradiation therapy has been the cornerstone for treating squamous cell carcinoma of the anal canal,[59–61] whereas surgery is now typically reserved for patients with local failure after chemoradiation. Compared with CT, PET/CT has been shown to have higher sensitivity (91% vs 59%) in identifying primary anal tumors, and it could detect

17% of abnormal nodes previously missed by CT and physical examination.[62] Furthermore, post-therapy FDG-PET has been found to be predictive of progression-free and cause-specific survival after chemoradiation therapy for anal cancer.[63] Compared with studies on rectal cancer, however, those concerning the impact of PET/CT on treatment planning of anal cancer are even more sparse, partly due to the rarity of the disease.[57,64–68]

The largest study on FDG-PET and anal cancer was conducted by Winton and colleagues,[65] in which the investigators evaluated the use of FDG-PET on nodal staging, radiation planning, and disease prognosis of 61 patients with squamous cell carcinoma of the anus. The patients underwent different combinations of conventional tumor staging methods (digital rectal examination, examination under anesthesia, endorectal ultrasound, CT, and MR imaging) followed by PET or PET/CT. Changes of stage occurred in 14 of 61 patients (23%), with 9 patients (15%) upstaged and 5 patients (8%) downstaged. More frequent changes in tumor stage were observed in tumors with more advanced T stage. Of the 22 patients with initial T1 stage, 3 (14%) had a change in nodal stage after PET, whereas 10 of 24 patients (42%) with T2 stage and 6 of 16 (38%) patients with T3/4 tumors had altered nodal stage after PET. PET was validated by biopsy as correct whenever there were discrepancies between PET and conventional staging for metastatic disease.

The study by de Winton and colleagues[65] also showed a significant change of treatment planning after the addition of PET. The treatment intent was changed in 2 of 61 patients (3%) and the radiotherapy field was changed to cover or exclude nodal disease in 8 (13%) patients. Prognoses also differed depending on the staging methods. Patients with PET-staged N2/3 disease had a 70% progression-free survival whereas those with N2/3 stage based on conventional staging methods had approximately 55% progression-free survival.

Additionally, a study conducted by Nguyen and colleagues[67] supported the notion that FDG-PET can help anal cancer radiation therapy planning. PET altered treatment planning in 11 of 48 patients (19%) due to identification of additional nodal involvement.[67] A small series also showed that integration of PET changed PTV in 1 of 3 patients with anal carcinoma.[57] It is difficult to draw any conclusion, however, from a study of only 3 patients.

Mai and colleagues[66] further investigated whether or not it was safe to reduce radiation doses to CT-enlarged but FDG-PET–negative

inguinal nodes. Among 36 patients, 16 suspicious inguinal nodes from 9 patients were identified by CT but only 3 nodes from 3 patients were PET positive. Consequently, radiation doses to the inguinal nodes were reduced from 50.4 to 54 Gy to 36 Gy for the 6 patients with CT-enlarged but PET-negative nodes. During the 3-year follow-up period, there was no disease recurrence in the inguinal lymph nodes in all patients, including those who received reduced radiation dose due to negative PET findings. Thus, it seemed that reduction of the irradiation dose to CT-enlarged but PET-negative inguinal nodes among anal cancer patients did not lead to increased local failure, although the results should be interpreted with caution given the small sample size and short follow-up period.

Overall, the few studies all showed promising results of using FDG-PET to aid radiation planning, either by identifying previously undetected disease or preventing unnecessary dose to PET-negative sites. Integrating PET in radiation treatment decision making could be feasible and potentially beneficial given its high sensitivity and specificity in delineating target structures and predicting treatment response.

SUMMARY

The use of PET/CT in radiation treatment planning has the potential to improve tumor volume delineation, reduce geographic misses, and decrease treatment-related toxicities in some cancers of the gastrointestinal tract. Data for esophageal cancer are abundant and they support the notion that PET/CT can have an impact on tumor volume definition. Although similar findings are also observed in rectal cancer, changes in tumor volume delineation may not always have a major impact on the overall radiation field because the typical radiation fields for rectal cancer also encompass pelvic nodal regions. For anal cancer, although limited results are available, existing data suggest that possible benefits of FDG-PET could include coverage of additional nodal disease and avoidance of excessive radiation to PET-negative sites. Virtually no data exist on how PET/CT might have any advantage over CT in radiation treatment planning for pancreatic cancer; there has also been no study concerning the use of PET/CT in radiation treatment planning for gastric cancer. Although many studies suggest that PET/CT may affect tumor volume and nodal delineation, studies correlating pathologic evaluation with PET/CT findings are necessary to firmly establish the role of PET/CT in radiotherapy planning. Moreover, the influence of PET/CT-based radiation treatment planning on treatment outcome has not been addressed. Hence, long-term follow-up is warranted to determine the impact of PET/CT-based radiation therapy on local control, patterns of failure, and treatment-related toxicity. Finally, cost-effectiveness studies also are needed to examine the economic impact of PET/CT in radiation therapy planning.

REFERENCES

1. Deniaud-Alexandre E, Touboul E, Lerouge D, et al. Impact of computed tomography and 18F-deoxy-glucose coincidence detection emission tomography image fusion for optimization of conformal radiotherapy in non-small-cell lung cancer. Int J Radiat Oncol Biol Phys 2005;63(5):1432–41.

2. Bradley J, Thorstad WL, Mutic S, et al. Impact of FDG-PET on radiation therapy volume delineation in non-small-cell lung cancer. Int J Radiat Oncol Biol Phys 2004;59(1):78–86.

3. Ashamalla H, Rafla S, Parikh K, et al. The contribution of integrated PET/CT to the evolving definition of treatment volumes in radiation treatment planning in lung cancer. Int J Radiat Oncol Biol Phys 2005; 63(4):1016–23.

4. Moule RN, Kayani I, Mouddin SA, et al. The potential advantages of (18)FDG PET/CT-based target volume delineation in radiotherapy planning of head and neck cancer. Radiother Oncol 2010; 97(2):189–93.

5. Vila A, Sanchez-Reyes A, Conill C, et al. Comparison of positron emission tomography (PET) and computed tomography (CT) for better target volume definition in radiation therapy planning. Clin Transl Oncol 2010;12(5):367–73.

6. Okubo M, Nishimura Y, Nakamatsu K, et al. Radiation treatment planning using positron emission and computed tomography for lung and pharyngeal cancers: a multiple-threshold method for [(18)F] fluoro-2-deoxyglucose activity. Int J Radiat Oncol Biol Phys 2010;77(2):350–6.

7. Razfar A, Heron DE, Branstetter BF, et al. Positron emission tomography-computed tomography adds to the management of salivary gland malignancies. Laryngoscope 2010;120(4):734–8.

8. Ciernik IF, Dizendorf E, Baumert BG, et al. Radiation treatment planning with an integrated positron emission and computer tomography (PET/CT): a feasibility study. Int J Radiat Oncol Biol Phys 2003; 57(3):853–63.

9. Gondi V, Bradley K, Mehta M, et al. Impact of hybrid fluorodeoxyglucose positron-emission tomography/computed tomography on radiotherapy planning in esophageal and non-small-cell lung cancer. Int J Radiat Oncol Biol Phys 2007;67(1):187–95.

10. Ashamalla H, Guirgius A, Bieniek E, et al. The impact of positron emission tomography/computed tomography in edge delineation of gross tumor volume for head and neck cancers. Int J Radiat Oncol Biol Phys 2007;68(2):388–95.

11. Weber WA. Positron emission tomography as an imaging biomarker. J Clin Oncol 2006;24(20): 3282–92.

12. Hillner BE, Siegel BA, Shields AF, et al. The impact of positron emission tomography (PET) on expected management during cancer treatment: findings of the National Oncologic PET registry. Cancer 2009; 115(2):410–8.

13. Leong T, Everitt C, Yuen K, et al. A prospective study to evaluate the impact of FDG-PET on CT-based radiotherapy treatment planning for oesophageal cancer. Radiother Oncol 2006;78(3):254–61.

14. Kim K, Park SJ, Kim BT, et al. Evaluation of lymph node metastases in squamous cell carcinoma of the esophagus with positron emission tomography. Ann Thorac Surg 2001;71(1):290–4.

15. Meltzer CC, Luketich JD, Friedman D, et al. Whole-body FDG positron emission tomographic imaging for staging esophageal cancer comparison with computed tomography. Clin Nucl Med 2000; 25(11):882–7.

16. Choi JY, Lee KH, Shim YM, et al. Improved detection of individual nodal involvement in squamous cell carcinoma of the esophagus by FDG PET. J Nucl Med 2000;41(5):808–15.

17. van Westreenen HL, Heeren PA, van Dullemen HM, et al. Positron emission tomography with F-18-fluoro-deoxyglucose in a combined staging strategy of esophageal cancer prevents unnecessary surgical explorations. J Gastrointest Surg 2005;9(1):54–61.

18. Rasanen JV, Sihvo EI, Knuuti MJ, et al. Prospective analysis of accuracy of positron emission tomography, computed tomography, and endoscopic ultrasonography in staging of adenocarcinoma of the esophagus and the esophagogastric junction. Ann Surg Oncol 2003;10(8):954–60.

19. Luketich JD, Schauer PR, Meltzer CC, et al. Role of positron emission tomography in staging esophageal cancer. Ann Thorac Surg 1997;64(3):765–9.

20. Schreurs LM, Busz DM, Paardekooper GM, et al. Impact of 18-fluorodeoxyglucose positron emission tomography on computed tomography defined target volumes in radiation treatment planning of esophageal cancer: reduction in geographic misses with equal inter-observer variability*. Dis Esophagus 2010;23(6):493–501.

21. Shimizu S, Hosokawa M, Itoh K, et al. Can hybrid FDG-PET/CT detect subclinical lymph node metastasis of esophageal cancer appropriately and contribute to radiation treatment planning? A comparison of image-based and pathological findings. Int J Clin Oncol 2009;14(5):421–5.

22. Muijs CT, Schreurs LM, Busz DM, et al. Consequences of additional use of PET information for target volume delineation and radiotherapy dose distribution for esophageal cancer. Radiother Oncol 2009;93(3):447–53.

23. MacManus M, Nestle U, Rosenzweig KE, et al. Use of PET and PET/CT for radiation therapy planning: IAEA expert report 2006–2007. Radiother Oncol 2009;91(1):85–94.

24. Schreurs LM, Pultrum BB, Koopmans KP, et al. Better assessment of nodal metastases by PET/CT fusion compared to side-by-side PET/CT in oesophageal cancer. Anticancer Res 2008;28(3B): 1867–73.

25. Hong TS, Killoran JH, Mamede M, et al. Impact of manual and automated interpretation of fused PET/CT data on esophageal target definitions in radiation planning. Int J Radiat Oncol Biol Phys 2008;72(5): 1612–8.

26. Moureau-Zabotto L, Touboul E, Lerouge D, et al. Impact of CT and 18F-deoxyglucose positron emission tomography image fusion for conformal radiotherapy in esophageal carcinoma. Int J Radiat Oncol Biol Phys 2005;63(2):340–5.

27. Vali FS, Nagda S, Hall W, et al. Comparison of standardized uptake value-based positron emission tomography and computed tomography target volumes in esophageal cancer patients undergoing radiotherapy. Int J Radiat Oncol Biol Phys 2010; 78(4):1057–63.

28. Vesprini D, Ung Y, Dinniwell R, et al. Improving observer variability in target delineation for gastro-oesophageal cancer—the role of (18F)fluoro-2-deoxy-D-glucose positron emission tomography/computed tomography. Clin Oncol (R Coll Radiol) 2008;20(8):631–8.

29. Konski A, Doss M, Milestone B, et al. The integration of 18-fluoro-deoxy-glucose positron emission tomography and endoscopic ultrasound in the treatment-planning process for esophageal carcinoma. Int J Radiat Oncol Biol Phys 2005;61(4): 1123–8.

30. Vrieze O, Haustermans K, De Wever W, et al. Is there a role for FGD-PET in radiotherapy planning in esophageal carcinoma? Radiother Oncol 2004; 73(3):269–75.

31. Yu W, Fu XL, Zhang YJ, et al. GTV spatial conformity between different delineation methods by 18FDG PET/CT and pathology in esophageal cancer. Radiother Oncol 2009;93(3):441–6.

32. Russo S, Butler J, Ove R, et al. Locally advanced pancreatic cancer: a review. Semin Oncol 2007; 34(4):327–34.

33. Willett CG, Czito BG, Bendell JC, et al. Locally advanced pancreatic cancer. J Clin Oncol 2005; 23(20):4538–44.

34. Kitajima K, Murakami K, Yamasaki E, et al. Performance of integrated FDG-PET/Contrast-enhanced CT in the diagnosis of recurrent pancreatic cancer: comparison with integrated FDG-PET/Non-contrast-enhanced CT and enhanced CT. Mol Imaging Biol 2009;12(4):452–9.

35. Lachter J, Adler AC, Keidar Z, et al. FDG-PET/CT identifies a curable pancreatic cancer surgical tract metastasis after failure by other imaging modalities. Isr Med Assoc J 2008;10(3):243–4.

36. Antoch G, Saoudi N, Kuehl H, et al. Accuracy of whole-body dual-modality fluorine-18-2-fluoro-2-deoxy-D-glucose positron emission tomography and computed tomography (FDG-PET/CT) for tumor staging in solid tumors: comparison with CT and PET. J Clin Oncol 2004;22(21):4357–68.

37. Kantorova I, Lipska L, Belohlavek O, et al. Routine (18)F-FDG PET preoperative staging of colorectal cancer: comparison with conventional staging and its impact on treatment decision making. J Nucl Med 2003;44(11):1784–8.

38. Topkan E, Yavuz AA, Aydin M, et al. Comparison of CT and PET-CT based planning of radiation therapy in locally advanced pancreatic carcinoma. J Exp Clin Cancer Res 2008;27:41.

39. Seo Y, Kim MS, Yoo S, et al. Stereotactic body radiation therapy boost in locally advanced pancreatic cancer. Int J Radiat Oncol Biol Phys 2009;75(5): 1456–61.

40. Crane CH, Willett CG. Stereotactic radiotherapy for pancreatic cancer? Cancer 2009;115(3):468–72.

41. Hoyer M, Roed H, Sengelov L, et al. Phase-II study on stereotactic radiotherapy of locally advanced pancreatic carcinoma. Radiother Oncol 2005;76(1): 48–53.

42. Schellenberg D, Goodman KA, Lee F, et al. Gemcitabine chemotherapy and single-fraction stereotactic body radiotherapy for locally advanced pancreatic cancer. Int J Radiat Oncol Biol Phys 2008;72(3):678–86.

43. Schellenberg D, Quon A, Minn AY, et al. (18)Fluoro-deoxyglucose PET is prognostic of progression-free and overall survival in locally advanced pancreas cancer treated with stereotactic radiotherapy. Int J Radiat Oncol Biol Phys 2010;77(5):1420–5.

44. Delbeke D, Martin WH. PET and PET-CT for evaluation of colorectal carcinoma. Semin Nucl Med 2004;34(3):209–23.

45. Capirci C, Rampin L, Erba PA, et al. Sequential FDG-PET/CT reliably predicts response of locally advanced rectal cancer to neo-adjuvant chemo-radiation therapy. Eur J Nucl Med Mol Imaging 2007;34(10):1583–93.

46. Cascini GL, Avallone A, Delrio P, et al. 18F-FDG PET is an early predictor of pathologic tumor response to preoperative radiochemotherapy in locally

advanced rectal cancer. J Nucl Med 2006;47(8): 1241–8.

47. Denecke T, Rau B, Hoffmann KT, et al. Comparison of CT, MRI and FDG-PET in response prediction of patients with locally advanced rectal cancer after multimodal preoperative therapy: is there a benefit in using functional imaging? Eur Radiol 2005;15(8): 1658–66.

48. Elstrom RL, Leonard JP, Coleman M, et al. Combined PET and low-dose, noncontrast CT scanning obviates the need for additional diagnostic contrast-enhanced CT scans in patients undergoing staging or restaging for lymphoma. Ann Oncol 2008; 19(10):1770–3.

49. Calvo FA, Domper M, Matute R, et al. 18F-FDG positron emission tomography staging and restaging in rectal cancer treated with preoperative chemoradiation. Int J Radiat Oncol Biol Phys 2004;58(2):528–35.

50. Capirci C, Rubello D, Pasini F, et al. The role of dual-time combined 18-fluorodeoxyglucose positron emission tomography and computed tomography in the staging and restaging workup of locally advanced rectal cancer, treated with preoperative chemoradiation therapy and radical surgery. Int J Radiat Oncol Biol Phys 2009;74(5):1461–9.

51. Gearhart SL, Frassica D, Rosen R, et al. Improved staging with pretreatment positron emission tomography/computed tomography in low rectal cancer. Ann Surg Oncol 2006;13(3):397–404.

52. Abdel-Nabi H, Doerr RJ, Lamonica DM, et al. Staging of primary colorectal carcinomas with fluorine-18 fluorodeoxyglucose whole-body PET: correlation with histopathologic and CT findings. Radiology 1998;206(3):755–60.

53. Bassi MC, Turri L, Sacchetti G, et al. FDG-PET/CT imaging for staging and target volume delineation in preoperative conformal radiotherapy of rectal cancer. Int J Radiat Oncol Biol Phy 2008;70(5): 1423–6.

54. Paskeviciute B, Bolling T, Brinkmann M, et al. Impact of (18)F-FDG-PET/CT on staging and irradiation of patients with locally advanced rectal cancer. Strahlenther Onkol 2009;185(4):260–5.

55. Ciernik IF, Huser M, Burger C, et al. Automated functional image-guided radiation treatment planning for rectal cancer. Int J Radiat Oncol Biol Phys 2005; 62(3):893–900.

56. Patel DA, Chang ST, Goodman KA, et al. Impact of integrated PET/CT on variability of target volume delineation in rectal cancer. Technol Cancer Res Treat 2007;6(1):31–6.

57. Anderson C, Koshy M, Staley C, et al. PET-CT fusion in radiation management of patients with anorectal tumors. Int J Radiat Oncol Biol Phys 2007;69(1): 155–62.

58. Roels S, Slagmolen P, Nuyts J, et al. Biological image-guided radiotherapy in rectal cancer: challenges and pitfalls. Int J Radiat Oncol Biol Phys 2009;75(3):782–90.

59. Nigro ND, Vaitkevicius VK, Considine B Jr. Combined therapy for cancer of the anal canal: a preliminary report. 1974. Dis Colon Rectum 1993;36(7):709–11.

60. Flam M, John M, Pajak TF, et al. Role of mitomycin in combination with fluorouracil and radiotherapy, and of salvage chemoradiation in the definitive nonsurgical treatment of epidermoid carcinoma of the anal canal: results of a phase III randomized intergroup study. J Clin Oncol 1996;14(9):2527–39.

61. Bartelink H, Roelofsen F, Eschwege F, et al. Concomitant radiotherapy and chemotherapy is superior to radiotherapy alone in the treatment of locally advanced anal cancer: results of a phase III randomized trial of the European organization for research and treatment of cancer radiotherapy and gastrointestinal cooperative Groups. J Clin Oncol 1997;15(5):2040–9.

62. Cotter SE, Grigsby PW, Siegel BA, et al. FDG-PET/CT in the evaluation of anal carcinoma. Int J Radiat Oncol Biol Phys 2006;65(3):720–5.

63. Schwarz JK, Siegel BA, Dehdashti F, et al. Tumor response and survival predicted by post-therapy FDG-PET/CT in anal cancer. Int J Radiat Oncol Biol Phys 2008;71(1):180–6.

64. Day E, Betler J, Parda D, et al. A region growing method for tumor volume segmentation on PET images for rectal and anal cancer patients. Med Phys 2009;36(10):4349–58.

65. Winton E, Heriot AG, Ng M, et al. The impact of 18-fluorodeoxyglucose positron emission tomography on the staging, management and outcome of anal cancer. Br J Cancer 2009;100(5):693–700.

66. Mai SK, Welzel G, Hermann B, et al. Can the radiation dose to CT-enlarged but FDG-PET-negative inguinal lymph nodes in anal cancer be reduced? Strahlenther Onkol 2009;185(4):254–9.

67. Nguyen BT, Joon DL, Khoo V, et al. Assessing the impact of FDG-PET in the management of anal cancer. Radiother Oncol 2008;87(3):376–82.

68. Pepek JM, Willett CG, Czito BG. Radiation therapy advances for treatment of anal cancer. J Natl Compr Canc Netw 2010;8(1):123–9.

The Role of Functional Imaging in Radiotherapy Planning and Management for Gynecologic Malignancies

Daniel J. Ma, MD[a], Susan Guo, MD[b], Shetal N. Shah, MD[c], Shyam M. Srinivas, MD, PhD[d], Roger M. Macklis, MD[b],*

KEYWORDS

- Gynecologic malignancies • Cervical cancer
- Endometrial cancer • Functional imaging

As is the case for many other clinical areas, the role of ionizing radiation in the management of gynecologic (GYN) tumors is currently under revision based on new technologies and on new details relating to long-term treatment toxicities. Convincing evidence for a curative role for radiotherapy in GYN malignancies dates from the early 20th century. Over time, many reasonably well-defined algorithms for tumor management have been codified and validated. For both cervical and endometrial cancer, the core of the clinical problem often involves a strong concern over local control in addition to concerns about distant metastatic disease. This local control mandate prompts tumor management algorithms heavily focused on anatomic modalities such as surgery and local radiotherapy. In some cases, systemic cytotoxic therapy and hormonal treatments also play important but secondary roles. In attempting to define the exact location of tumor target sites, the historical reliance on 2-dimensional (2D) imaging has now been replaced with 3D and even 4D volumetric imaging sequences capable of describing the precise anatomic relationships with respect to sensitive normal tissues and dynamic target localization.

In addition to allowing much greater technical precision, the modern era also allows investigation of target physiology and it is the potential incorporation of physiologic information into the treatment-planning rubric that gives modern PET-CT its allure and promise. Although oncologic PET scanning has now been clinically available for more than 10 years, it is only recently that sufficient investigative and retrospective data have become available to confidently assert that future radiotherapy treatment planning will include functional imaging as an useful dimension of clinical characterization for most GYN tumors.

[a] Department of Radiation Oncology, Mallinckrodt Institute of Radiology, Siteman Cancer Center, Washington University Medical Center, 4921 Parkview Place, St Louis, MO 63110, USA
[b] Department of Radiation Oncology, Cleveland Clinic Lerner College of Medicine and Taussig Cancer Center, 9500 Euclid Avenue, Cleveland, OH 44195, USA
[c] Departments of Abdominal Imaging and Nuclear Medicine, Center for PET and Molecular Imaging, Imaging Institute, Cleveland Clinic, Cleveland, OH, USA
[d] Department of Nuclear Medicine, Center for PET and Molecular Imaging, Imaging Institute, Cleveland Clinic, Cleveland, OH, USA
* Corresponding author.
E-mail address: macklir@ccf.org

PET Clin 6 (2011) 195–205
doi:10.1016/j.cpet.2011.02.006

CERVICAL CANCER
Introduction

Invasive cervical cancer is the third most common gynecologic malignancy in the United States. It is the fifth leading cause of cancer deaths in women ages 35 to 54 years and is therefore a leading cause of lives lost.[1] Cervical cancer confined to the lower pelvis can be cured by surgery or chemoradiotherapy.[2] Many well-known pretreatment prognostic factors exist, including clinical staging, tumor diameter, and tumor volume.[3-5] Nevertheless, the ability to evaluate these prognostic factors may be limited using traditional examination techniques. Compared with surgical staging, clinical staging as defined by the International Federation of Gynecology and Obstetrics (FIGO) has been shown to understage up to 20% to 30% of stage IB patients, and up to 64% of stage IIIB patients.[6] Traditional examination techniques may lead to inadequate treatment decisions because of a misdiagnosis of a patient's true disease burden (**Fig. 1**).

Because of the limitations of traditional examination techniques, imaging techniques have been proposed as adjuncts to clinical examination for treatment planning. Computed tomography (CT) imaging with and without intravenous contrast has been investigated for staging cervical cancer. The accuracy of CT scans for staging the primary tumor has been found to be between 63% and 88%.[7] When used for detecting involved lymph nodes, CT scans have an accuracy of 77% to 85%.[8] However, because of its reliance on size criteria for detecting involved nodes, CT scans have only a 25% sensitivity for histologically positive nodes.[9] When compared with CT imaging, magnetic resonance imaging (MR imaging) offers improved soft tissue contrast. As a result, MR imaging can predict endometrial involvement in about 84% to 96% of cases, as opposed to 55% to 80% by CT, and has a high negative predictive value (NPV).[10,11] Although para-aortic nodal metastasis can be detected with high specificity, the sensitivity is low at only 50%.[12] Furthermore, T2-weighted MR imaging of cervical tumors often contains a so-called "gray zone" of uncertain clinical significance surrounding the tumor.[13] Thus, it may be difficult to delineate tumor boundaries based on T2-MR imaging.

Improvements in tumor delineation and staging by functional imaging modalities such as PET can improve treatment decisions and increase the precision of targeted radiotherapy.[14,15] In addition, multiple investigative radioactive tracers exist for PET scanning, allowing clinicians to image a variety of cellular processes ranging from proliferation to

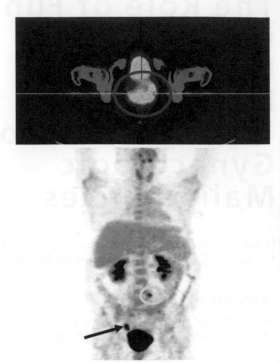

Fig. 1. Cervical cancer upstaged by initial PET-CT. Images are of a 48-year-old woman with diagnosis of squamous cell carcinoma of the cervix. Fused PET/CT was obtained for initial staging. Fused axial PET/CT (*upper*) and volumetric MIP (*lower*) images demonstrate abnormal FDG uptake in the cervix from cervical carcinoma (*red circle*). Note an 8-mm FDG-avid left para-aortic metastatic lymph node (*yellow circle*), unenlarged by CT criteria. Distal right ureteral activity (*blue arrow* in volumetric MIP image) as well as physiologic ovarian FDG uptake can be pitfalls in PET imaging of the pelvis.

hypoxia. Nevertheless, PET lacks the spatial resolution present in anatomic imaging modalities such as MR imaging.[16] Therefore, radiation treatment planning based on PET requires a careful assessment of the modality's strengths and limitations. This section will explore the issues of using PET for radiation treatment planning in cervical cancer. As fluorodeoxyglucose (FDG) is the most prevalent radiotracer in use, most of this text will cover the literature concerning FDG-PET.

Histologic Dependence

Before a full discussion on FDG-PET treatment planning can begin, one must first acknowledge that a relationship may exist between cervical cancer histology and FDG uptake. Because of the correspondence between FDG-avidity and glycolytic activity, one can hypothesize that FDG uptake might be linked with tumor histology. This would be significant, as many proposed PET segmentation and prognostic techniques involve using the standardized uptake value (SUV) of a particular tumor. If a difference between mean or maximum SUV values among differing tumor histologies exists, different SUV treatment planning algorithms may be required for different tumor histologies.

Differences in FDG uptake among different histologic types was first observed in non–small-cell lung cancer (NSCLC). Various groups have demonstrated that FDG uptake in NSCLC is significantly different between adenocarcinomas versus squamous cell carcinomas, and between degrees of tumor differentiation.[17–20] Similar findings have now been demonstrated in cervical cancer. In a study of 240 patients with cervical cancer, mean SUV value was found to be significantly different among squamous cell carcinoma (mean SUV 11.91), adenosquamous carcinoma (mean SUV 8.85), and adenocarcinoma (mean SUV 8.05) histologies.[21] This same study also found a significant correlation between SUV values and cervical cancer grade, with higher SUV values correlated with more poorly differentiated tumors.

The application of this finding to other publications on FDG-PET in cervical cancer is somewhat problematic. As this finding was not reported until 2009, most of the studies cited within this article were performed on a mixed population of different cervical histologies and grades. Approximately 85% of cervical cancers are squamous cell carcinomas, so it is unclear if the small population of adenosquamous carcinomas and adenocarcinomas within these studies would substantially affect results.[22] In the very least, future studies should be cognizant of the possible confounding effect of cervical cancer histology on FDG uptake and stratify results accordingly.

Nodal Staging and Treatment Implications

Because of the limitations of CT and MR imaging scans in detecting histologically positive nodes, various groups have investigated the efficacy of FDG-PET in improving nodal staging. In a meta-analysis of lymph node detection by FDG-PET, MR imaging, and CT, FDG-PET was found to be superior to both of the anatomic imaging methods.[23] Studies comparing lymph node dissection to FDG-PET suggest that the sensitivity of FDG-PET in detecting nodal metastases is dependent on the clinical stage. For patients with clinical Ib1 or Ib2 disease, the sensitivity for detecting pelvic lymph nodes is only 30% to 50%.[24,25] For more advanced disease, the sensitivity for detecting both pelvic and para-aortic

nodal disease climbs to the order of 90%.[26] This stage dependence is likely attributable to an increasing volume of tumor deposits within lymph nodes with higher stage. One study reported a size-dependence in the sensitivity for detecting lymph nodes in patients with early stage cervical cancer. The sensitivity was 52% for nodes larger than 5 mm and rose to 65% for nodes larger than 1 cm.[27] Nevertheless, as size criteria for anatomic imaging like CT or MR might mistakenly dismiss any node smaller than 1 cm, one could still view the 52% to 65% sensitivity rate of FDG-PET for nodes smaller than 1 cm as an improvement (Fig. 2).

The identification of FDG-avid lymph nodes is important because it has a relationship to a patient's prognosis. In a study retrospectively analyzing the pretreatment staging PETs on 560 patients receiving surgery alone, surgery plus

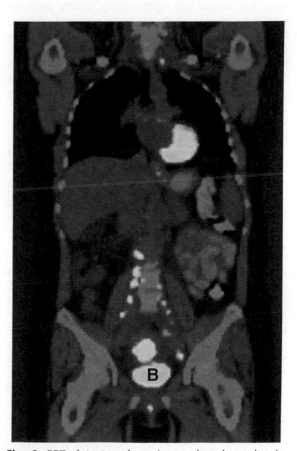

Fig. 2. PET detects subcentimeter lymph nodes in a 49-year-old woman with squamous cell cervical cancer: initial staging. PET primary tumor SUV_{max} and presence of retroperitoneal nodes are independent prognosticators (but not addressed by FIGO staging scheme). Conventional imaging lacks sensitivity of pathologic subcentimeter nodes.

postoperative radiation, or definitive radiation with or without chemotherapy, 47% of patients were found to have PET-positive nodes at diagnosis.[28] Additionally, the extent of lymph node involvement on PET stratified patients into distinct outcome groups. The presence of PET-positive pelvic lymph nodes yielded a harm ratio of 2.40 for disease-specific survival relative to node-negative patients, whereas the presence of para-aortic nodes yielded a harm ratio of 5.88. Supraclavicular lymph node involvement had the highest harm ratio at 30.27.

Detecting nodal metastases also has implications for a patient's treatment. Early-stage patients who would have otherwise received surgical intervention may be treated with concurrent chemoradiation.[29] Patients with para-aortic lymph node involvement may benefit from the use of extended radiation treatment fields, although at the cost of increased morbidity.[30] FDG-PET may also be useful for determining which patients would require concurrent cisplatin-based chemotherapy with radiation therapy. In a prospective data registry of 65 patients with cervical cancer and PET-negative lymph nodes, no difference in 5-year cause-specific survival was found between patients receiving concurrent chemoradiation and patients receiving definitive radiation alone.[31] However, the chemoradiation group had a higher rate of pelvic and hematologic complications. Although studies such as these should be verified in the context of a prospective, randomized trial, it does suggest the possibility of using FDG-PET as a future tool for triaging patients with cervical cancer for directed interventions.

Primary Tumor Staging

As a functional rather than anatomic imaging modality, defining tumor borders by FDG-PET has inherent difficulties. For example, PET is not an effective method for detecting parametrial disease extension without correlating the image with anatomic imaging.[32] Furthermore, defining reproducible tumor volumes using SUV values requires strict guidelines for image acquisition, including injection time, activity injected, blood glucose level, acquisition time, and Foley catheter placement. After standardizing these variables, however, some institutions have had success in developing algorithms for generating a so-called "metabolic tumor volume" (MTV). Investigations have generally focused on SUV thresholding techniques that create isocontours based on a set percentage of the maximum SUV value. Using this technique, one group compared tumor diameter as defined by CT with varying SUV thresholds in 51 patients with cervical cancer (91% squamous cell). In this study, the tumor volume as defined by the 40% threshold from SUV_{max} was found to be the best fit to the tumor volume as defined by CT.[33] This SUV threshold of 40% was subsequently validated in a series of 41 patients with early-stage cervical cancer who underwent pretreatment FDG-PET and subsequent surgery. Using this threshold, the FDG-PET tumor diameter measurement was correlated with the pathologic tumor diameter in the surgical specimen with a coefficient of determination of 0.951 and a correlation coefficient of 0.757.[34] Work on PET autosegmentation continues to be an active area of research and many promising algorithms involving region growing and edge detection continue to be developed.[35]

Radiation Treatment Planning: External Beam

Decisions regarding treating patients with cervical cancer with external beam irradiation involve considering the volume to be irradiated and the irradiation dose. The irradiated volume includes either the pelvis only or the pelvis and para-aortic regions.[36] Although evaluation of pelvic nodes by PET/CT does not necessarily modify the therapeutic volume for the pelvis (which will be given external beam radiation regardless), para-aortic foci of pathologic uptake on PET/CT may influence treatment portals.[37] In the era of intensity modulated radiation therapy (IMRT), it may be possible to boost the radiation dose to FDG-avid lymph nodes as well. In a series of 208 patients, lymph nodes were scored as either positive or negative by PET, and lymph node size was measured by CT. Lymph node irradiation dose and sites of failure were recorded. For PET-negative nodes smaller than 1 cm that received 66.8 Gy, there were 0 of 76 nodal site failures; however, PET-positive nodes smaller than 1 cm, receiving 66.8 Gy, had 3 out of 89 nodal site failures.[38] Furthermore, with proper IMRT planning, dose escalation to FDG-avid pelvic nodes need not come at higher doses to bowel and bladder.[39]

This PET/CT-based IMRT strategy has been successfully implemented in several institutions. At the Mallinckrodt Institute of Radiology (MIR), for example, PET/CT-based radiation planning is routinely used. Patients must first undergo a PET/CT radiotherapy simulation. The simulation is performed on a PET/CT scanner with the patient in the treatment position and uses standard fiducial markers and immobilization devices.[40] An MTV cervix is auto-segmented using the 40% SUV_{max} threshold technique as previously described. Pelvic vessels are also contoured and expanded to form a nodal target volume. These target volumes are further expanded as necessary to encompass FDG-avid lymph nodes (**Fig. 3**). Once the contours for the primary cervix tumor, the positive lymph nodes, and the regional lymph node volumes have been completed, the irradiation doses to the prescribed volumes can be planned using the radiotherapy treatment planning software. Published and validated correlative data suggesting choice of radiotherapy doses based on FDG-PET SUV levels are currently being acquired at many sites. At present, however, definitive dose/response data are largely lacking.

Using this PET/CT-guided IMRT strategy in conjunction with brachytherapy has yielded excellent results at MIR. In a prospective cohort of 452 patients with newly diagnosed cervical cancer treated with curative intent, patients treated with PET/CT-guided IMRT (n = 135) were compared with patients who were not treated with IMRT (n = 317).[41] Treatment involved external irradiation and brachytherapy, and 85% of patients received concurrent chemotherapy. With a mean follow-up of 52 months, there was improved disease-specific survival and overall survival in the PET/CT-guided IMRT cohort compared with the

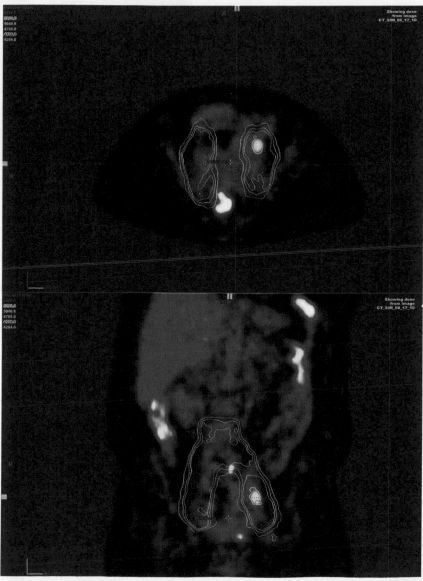

Fig. 3. External beam radiotherapy planning. PET can be used to define target volumes for external beam radiation. The FDG-avid left external iliac node is included in the target volume, as illustrated by the isodose curves.

non-IMRT cohort. Patients treated with PET/CT-guided IMRT also had a smaller rate of Grade 3 or greater bowel or bladder complications.

Radiation Treatment Planning: Brachytherapy

Intracavitary brachytherapy remains an essential component in definitive radiotherapy for cervical cancer. Traditional brachytherapy treatment planning is performed with 2D images from anterior-posterior and lateral radiographs. Three-dimensional image reconstruction and treatment planning is possible with CT, MR imaging, and FDG-PET. One of the advantages of 3D image–guided brachytherapy treatment planning is the ability to conform the target isodose surface to the gross and microscopic tumor volume by adjusting the dwell times and positions, which may potentially allow for decreased doses to the surrounding normal tissues as well.[42] However, the ability to perform 3D treatment planning for cervix cancer is predicated on the ability to accurately define the tumor volume.

In a prospective dosimetric study on 31 implants performed on 11 patients, dose distributions in a standard plan were compared with a plan allowing for more conformal coverage of the PET-defined volume. In this study, the dose to point A was higher with the optimized plans for both the first implant and the mid/last implants, whereas the dose to the bladder and rectum were not significantly different.[43] Thus, optimized treatment using PET allowed for improved dose to point A without significantly increasing the dose to normal tissues.

Prognosis and Prediction

It has long been known that persistent cervical tumor on clinical examination performed 1 to 3 months after completion of therapy is associated with an increased risk of recurrence and poor overall survival.[44] Furthermore, the early detection of residual disease may positively affect clinical outcome for selected patients.[45,46] However, assessment by clinical examination can be operator dependent and endophytic tumor morphologies do not lend themselves to easy examination.

The ability for FDG-PET to document metabolic response after chemoradiation therapy has been documented for a variety of clinical sites.[47–49] For cervical cancer, FDG-PET obtained only 3 months after the completion of therapy can be used to predict durable treatment response (**Fig. 4**).[50,51] In a prospective registry of patients with cervical cancer receiving definitive chemoradiotherapy, the presence of residual or progressive disease

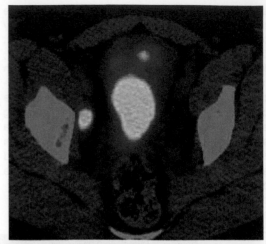
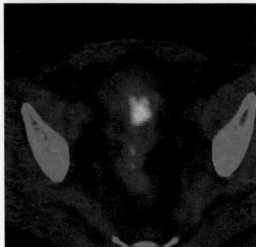

Fig. 4. PET/CT: cervical cancer monitoring therapy—residual posttreatment FDG avidity. Images are of a 36-year-old woman status post radiation therapy for cervical carcinoma (without extrapelvic disease). SUV$_{max}$ of primary tumor shows partial metabolic response associated with worse 5-year survival (32%) compared with complete metabolic response (80%) (P<.0001).

on FDG-PET 3 months after therapy was found to be more predictive of survival outcome than the pretreatment lymph node status.[52] FDG-PET is also useful for tracking the treatment response of cervical cancers during therapy, with a subset of patients achieving a complete metabolic response during radiotherapy.[53] Recommendations concerning the optimal timing of FDG-PET during and after radiotherapy will require further study, but currently 2 to 3 months is advised to allow time for radiation-induced inflammation to subside.

Research now suggests that pretreatment tumor metrics measured by FDG-PET may have prognostic significance as well. One retrospective review of 287 patients with stage IA2 through IVB cervical cancer found that SUV_{max} was a sensitive biomarker of treatment response and prognosis.[54] The overall survival rates at 5 years were 95% for an SUV_{max} of 5.2 or lower, 70% for an SUV_{max} greater than 5.2 but less than or equal to 13.3, and 44% for an SUV_{max} greater than 13.3. Further work by this group demonstrated that the intratumoral FDG metabolic heterogeneity on the pretreatment FDG-PET predicted risk of lymph node involvement at diagnosis, response to therapy, and risk of pelvic recurrence.[55] Work in developing these pretreatment FDG metrics into an imaging nomogram for patient stratification in clinical trials is currently under investigation.[56]

ENDOMETRIAL CANCER
Introduction

Endometrial cancer is the most common gynecologic malignancy in Western Europe and North America. The staging system is primarily surgical, with preoperative imaging to assess for the presence of systemic disease. However, in 20% of cases, clinical assessment and conventional preoperative imaging are incorrect in evaluating extent of disease.[57,58] Furthermore, the role of comprehensive surgical staging, including pelvic and para-aortic lymphadenectomy for all patients, is controversial. PET scans are being increasingly used to complement conventional imaging modalities to increase the accuracy of endometrial cancer staging. This is most commonly performed with the ^{18}F-FDG radiotracer. Fused PET/CT scans combine the anatomic detail provided by CT with metabolic information from FDG-PET.

Primary Tumor Staging

Studies examining the use of FDG-PET in staging primary endometrial tumors have reported modest sensitivities, ranging from 84.0% to 96.7%.[59–62] Suzuki and colleagues[59] examined 30 patients with endometrial cancer with FDG-PET, CT, and MR imaging, and concluded that FDG-PET was able to detect primary tumors with a higher sensitivity (96.7%) than CT/MR imaging (83.3%), although the difference was not statistically significant. Park and colleagues[61] analyzed 53 patients with uterine corpus tumors who underwent preoperative workup with imaging followed by surgical staging, and found comparable sensitivity, specificity, NPV, and positive predictive value (PPV) in PET/CT versus MR imaging. In this study, neither PET/CT nor MR imaging were able to detect very small focal lesions or thin, superficially spreading tumors. In another series, Picchio and colleagues[60]

reviewed the diagnostic accuracy of PET/CT in 32 patients with histologically proven endometrial cancer and correlated preoperative PET/CT findings with surgical specimens. Similar to Park and colleagues' analysis,[61] all the false negative lesions observed in this study were smaller than 1 cm.

Nodal Staging

Since 1988, the FIGO classification has recommended systemic pelvic and para-aortic lymphadenectomy for complete staging of endometrial cancer; however, prospective randomized trials have shown no survival benefit with lymphadenectomy.[63,64] CT and MR imaging have extensively been used to assess nodal spread of disease. A short-axis diameter of 10 mm or greater is accepted as the cutoff for suspicious nodal involvement. However, these imaging techniques have had reported low sensitivities of 20% to 65% and specificity of 73% to 99%.[65–70] FDG-PET has been studied as an additional noninvasive tool to identify patients who are at increased risk of nodal metastasis in hopes of avoiding the morbidities of lymphadenectomy in lower risk patients.

A prospective series of 20 patients by Horowitz and colleagues[62] showed a low sensitivity of 60% by lymph node regions. In the series of Picchio and colleagues,[60] 26 patients underwent lymphadenectomy. Nineteen had histologically negative nodes and 7 had histologically positive nodes. Of these 7 patients, 4 were correctly identified by PET/CT, yielding a sensitivity of 57.1%.[60] Histopathological analysis showed that lymph nodal lesion size was smaller than 1 cm in all 3 falsely negative patients. Kitajima and colleagues[71] reported a low PET/CT sensitivity in nodal detection, 53.3%, and correlated this to nodal size measured on CT. The detection rate for nodal metastasis was 66.7% for nodes between 5 and 9 mm and 16.7% for nodes smaller than 4 mm. Similarly, the analysis by Suzuki and colleagues[59] was unable to detect any of 5 cases of lymph node metastases smaller than 1 cm in diameter by FDG-PET. Because the mean value of spatial resolution of FDG-PET scanners is approximately 0.7 cm, small metastases in small lymph nodes are minimally detectable, making size an important limitation of using PET to characterize microscopic disease.[72–74] These series illustrate that the sensitivities of PET for lymph node staging have not yet been sufficient to replace lymphadenectomy.

The NPVs have consistently been high across multiple series reporting the use of FDG-PET for nodal-based analyses, ranging from 87.5% to 94.7% for para-aortic nodes and 80.8% to 98.9% for pelvic lymph nodes.[59,61] Two other series report overall nodal NPVs as 86.4% and 94.4%.[60,75] The investigators in these series suggest that pelvic lymphadenectomy may be spared in patients who are PET/CT negative, especially in poor surgical candidates with multiple comorbidities who cannot tolerate the additional toxicities of a lymph node dissection. This clinical hypothesis warrants further investigation in a prospective setting.

Distant Staging

In Picchio and colleagues' analysis,[60] 7 of 32 patients had PET/CT-positive findings for distant metastases.[60] This was validated by histopathological confirmation in 4 of the 7 cases and CT/MR confirmation in 3 of the 7 cases. PET/CT correctly identified distant metastases in all patients, yielding a sensitivity of 100%. The specificity was 96%. PPVs and NPVs were 87.5% and 100% respectively. Park and colleagues[61] reported comparable results with 100% sensitivity, 93.8% specificity, 62.5% PPV, and 100% NPV in their analysis of using PET/CT to evaluate distant metastases in 8 patients with distant sites of disease. The advantage of PET/CT over routine abdominal imaging is that PET/CT can encompass asymptomatic lesions that may not otherwise be detected. These findings suggest that the main benefit of PET/CT is to accurately detect, localize, and characterize distant metastases.

Variations with Tumor Grade

Tumor grade is an important prognostic factor in endometrial cancer. Low-grade endometrial carcinomas consist of moderately differentiated to well-differentiated endometrioid adenocarcinomas that arise within a background of endometrial hyperplasia. These tumors are often hormone sensitive and have a favorable prognosis. High-grade endometrial carcinomas are associated with endometrial atrophy and are not estrogen driven. These tumors are at high risk of relapse and metastatic disease.[76]

There is some evidence suggesting that FDG uptake correlates with tumor grade. In a study of 44 patients with endometrial cancer with PET scans conducted 2 weeks before surgery, the SUV_{max} of the primary tumor significantly correlated with tumor size, glucose transport-1 expression, and tumor grade.[77] Multivariate analysis revealed that of the 3, FIGO grade was the most significant factor associated with a maximum SUV greater than or equal to 17.6. The investigators proposed that the SUV_{max} of the primary tumor may be associated with aggressive biologic characteristics. However, other reports did not show correlation between FDG uptake and tumor grade.[61]

Estrogen Receptor Expression

Estrogen receptor (ER) expression coupled with glucose metabolism with radioactive tracer 16α-^{18}F-fluoro-17βestradiol (FES) has been used in functional PET, along with ^{18}F-FDG PET, in the differential diagnosis of benign and malignant uterine tumors.[78] Malignant tumors showed high glucose metabolism and low ER expression, whereas benign tumors showed low glucose metabolism and high ER expression.

Thirty-one patients with endometrial thickening or suspected malignancy underwent PET and MR imaging scans. Twenty-five of these patients were scanned before definitive surgery and 6 patients were scanned before whole-endometrium curettage.[79] Tumors were stratified into high-risk endometrial carcinoma (FIGO stage higher than Ib or histologic grade higher than grade 1), low-risk carcinoma (FIGO stage Ib or Ia and histologic grade 1), and endometrial hyperplasia. Patients with high-risk endometrial carcinoma had a significantly higher accumulation of ^{18}F-FDG than ^{18}F-FES, whereas patients with low-risk carcinoma did not show a significant difference in ^{18}F-FDG than in ^{18}F-FES uptake. Endometrial hyperplasia showed a significantly higher uptake for ^{18}F-FES than ^{18}F-FDG. The investigators reported that the ^{18}F-FDG to ^{18}F-FES ratio was significantly higher in high-risk carcinoma than low-risk carcinoma ($P<.01$) and endometrial hyperplasia ($P<.005$). Low-risk carcinoma also showed a significantly higher ^{18}F-FDG to ^{18}F-FES ratio than hyperplasia ($P<.0001$). An ^{18}F-FDG to ^{18}F-FES ratio of 2.0 provided 73% sensitivity and 100% specificity in distinguishing high-risk carcinoma from low-risk carcinoma. The investigators propose using this ratio as a noninvasive way to determine tumor aggressiveness, although they caution that their ratio cutoffs have not yet been evaluated in a prospective manner.

SUMMARY

FDG-PET and PET/CT have comparable sensitivities in staging primary endometrial lesions as conventional imaging modalities. The sensitivity is low for lymph node staging and is limited by the spatial resolution of PET, which cannot detect microscopic metastatic disease. FDG-PET staging should not replace surgical staging with lymphadenectomy. However, the high NPV of FDG-PET for nodal disease may allow selected patients who are poor surgical candidates to avoid morbidities of lymphadenectomy. FDG-PET is useful for accurately detecting the presence of distant metastases. In addition, FDG uptake can correlate with higher-grade tumors. Larger prospective studies are needed to clarify the role of FDG-PET and PET/CT in the preoperative evaluation of endometrial cancer.

REFERENCES

1. Jemal A, Murray T, Ward E, et al. Cancer statistics. CA Cancer J Clin 2005;2005(55):10–30.
2. Stehman F, Bundy B, DiSaia P, et al. Carcinoma of the cervix treated with irradiation therapy. I. A multivariate analysis of prognostic variables in the Gynecologic Oncology Group. Cancer 1991;67:2776–85.
3. FIGO. International Federation of Gynecology and Obstetrics: classification and staging of malignant tumors in the female pelvis: annual report on the results of treatment in gynecological cancer. Int J Gynaecol Obstet 1989;28:189.
4. Eifel PJ, Morris M, Wharton JT, et al. The influence of tumor size and morphology on the outcome of patients with FIGO stage IB squamous cell carcinoma of the uterine cervix. Int J Radiat Oncol Biol Phys 1994;29:9–16.
5. Garipagaoglu M, Tulunay G, Kose MF, et al. Prognostic factors in stage IB-IIA cervical carcinomas treated with postoperative radiotherapy. Eur J Gynaecol Oncol 1999;20:131–5.
6. Lagasse LD, Creasman WT, Shingleton HM, et al. Results and complications of operative staging in cervical cancer: experience of the Gynecologic Oncology Group. Gynecol Oncol 1980;9:90-8.
7. Kim SH, Han JK. Invasion of the urinary bladder by uterine cervical carcinoma: evaluation with MR imaging. AJR Am J Roentgenol 1997;168:393–406.
8. Hricak H, Hu KK. Radiology in invasive cervical cancer. AJR Am J Roentgenol 1996;167:1101.
9. Camilien L, Gordon D, Fruchter RG, et al. Predictive value of computerized tomography in the presurgical evaluation of primary carcinoma of the cervix. Gynecol Oncol 1988;30:209–15.
10. Hricak H, Lacey CG, Sandles LG, et al. Invasive cervical carcinoma: comparison of MR imaging and surgical findings. Radiology 1988;166:623–31.
11. Togashi K, Morikawa K, Kataoka ML, et al. Cervical cancer. J Magn Reson Imaging 1998;8:391–7.
12. Kim SH, Choi BI, Han JK, et al. Preoperative staging of uterine cervical carcinoma: comparison of CT and MRI in 99 patients. J Comput Assist Tomogr 1993;17:633–40.
13. Potter R, Haie-Meder C, Van Limbergen E, et al. Recommendations from gynaecological (GYN) GEC ESTRO working group (II): concepts and terms in 3D image-based treatment planning in cervix cancer brachytherapy-3D dose volume parameters and aspects of 3D image-based anatomy, radiation physics, radiobiology. Radiother Oncol 2006;78:67–77.
14. Soutter WP, Hanoch J, D'Arcy T, et al. Pretreatment tumour volume measurement on high-resolution magnetic resonance imaging as a predictor of survival in cervical cancer. BJOG 2004;111:741–7.
15. Grigsby PW, Siegel BA, Dehdashti F. Lymph node staging by positron emission tomography in patients with carcinoma of the cervix. J Clin Oncol 2001;19:3745–9.
16. Shibuya K, Yoshida E, Nishikido F, et al. Limit of spatial resolution in FDG-PET due to annihilation photon non-collinearity. World Congress on Medical Physics and Biomedical Engineering 2006. IFMBE Proceedings. 2007;14, Part 11:1667–71.
17. Kieninger AN, Welsh R, Bendick PJ, et al. Positron-emission tomography as a prognostic tool for early-stage lung cancer. Am J Surg 2006;191:433–6.
18. Vesselle H, Schmidt RA, Pugsley JM, et al. Lung cancer proliferation correlates with [F-18]fluorodeoxyglucose uptake by positron emission tomography. Clin Cancer Res 2000;6:3837–44.
19. de Geus-Oei LF, van Krieken JH, Aliredjo RP, et al. Biological correlates of FDG uptake in non-small cell lung cancer. Lung Cancer 2007;55:79–87.
20. Higashi K, Ueda Y, Seki H, et al. Fluorine-18-FDG PET imaging is negative in bronchioloalveolar lung carcinoma. J Nucl Med 1998;39:1016–20.
21. Kidd EA, Spencer CR, Huettner PC, et al. Cervical cancer histology and tumor differentiation affect 18F-fluorodeoxyglucose uptake. Cancer 2009;115(15):3548–54.
22. DeMay M. Practical principles of cytopathology. Revised edition. Chicago: American Society for Clinical Pathology Press; 2007. ISBN 978-0-89189-549-7.
23. Havrilesky LJ, Kulasingam SL, Matchar DB, et al. FDG-PET for management of cervical and ovarian cancer. Gynecol Oncol 2005;97:183–91.
24. Wright JD, Dehdashti F, Herzog TJ, et al. Preoperative lymph node staging of early-stage cervical carcinoma by [18F]-fluoro-2-deoxy-D-glucose-positron emission tomography. Cancer 2005;104(11):2484–91.
25. Yen TC, Ng KK, Ma SY, et al. Value of dual-phase 2-fluoro-2-deoxy-D-glucose positron emission tomography in cervical cancer. J Clin Oncol 2003;21(19):3651–8.
26. Rose PG, Adler LP, Rodriguez M, et al. Positron emission tomography for evaluating para-aortic nodal metastasis in locally advanced cervical cancer before surgical staging: a surgicopathologic study. J Clin Oncol 1999;17:41–5.
27. Roh JW, Seo SS, Lee S, et al. Role of positron emission tomography in pretreatment lymph node staging of uterine cervical cancer: a prospective

surgicopathologic correlation study. Eur J Cancer 2005;41:2086–92.

28. Kidd EA, Siegel BA, Dehdashti F, et al. Lymph node staging by positron emission tomography in cervical cancer: relationship to prognosis. J Clin Oncol 2010; 28(12):2108–13.

29. Pandharipande PV, Choy G, del Carmen MG, et al. MRI and PET/CT for triaging stage IB clinically operable cervical cancer to appropriate therapy: decision analysis to assess patient outcomes. Am J Roentgenol 2009;192(3):802–14.

30. Vigliotti AP, Wen BC, Hussey DH, et al. Extended field irradiation for carcinoma of the uterine cervix with positive periaortic nodes. Int J Radiat Oncol Biol Phys 1992;23:501–9.

31. Grigsby PW, Mutch DG, Rader J, et al. Lack of benefit of concurrent chemotherapy in patients with cervical cancer and negative lymph nodes by FDG–PET. Int J Radiat Oncol Biol Phys 2005;61: 444–9.

32. Park W, Park YJ, Huh SJ, et al. The usefulness of MRI and PET imaging for the detection of parametrial involvement and lymph node metastasis in patients with cervical cancer. Jpn J Clin Oncol 2005;35:260–4.

33. Miller TR, Grigsby PW. Measurement of tumor volume by PET to evaluate prognosis in patients with advanced cervical cancer treated by radiation therapy. Int J Radiat Oncol Biol Phys 2002;53(2): 353–9.

34. Showalter TN, Miller TR, Huettner P, et al. 18F-fluorodeoxyglucose-positron emission tomography and pathologic tumor size in early-stage invasive cervical cancer. Int J Gynecol Cancer 2009;19(8): 1412–4.

35. Zaidi H, El Naqa I. PET-guided delineation of radiation therapy treatment volumes: a survey of image segmentation techniques. Eur J Nucl Med Mol Imaging 2010;37(11):2165–87.

36. Grigsby PW. PET/CT imaging to guide cervical cancer therapy. Future Oncol 2009;5(7):953–8.

37. Magné N, Chargari C, Vicenzi L, et al. New trends in the evaluation and treatment of cervix cancer: the role of FDG-PET. Cancer Treat Rev 2008;34(8): 671–81.

38. Grigsby PW, Singh AK, Siegel BA, et al. Lymph node control in cervical cancer. Int J Radiat Oncol Biol Phys 2004;59(3):706–12.

39. Esthappan J, Mutic S, Malyapa RS, et al. Treatment planning guidelines regarding the use of CT/PET-guided IMRT for cervical carcinoma with positive paraaortic lymph nodes. Int J Radiat Oncol Biol Phys 2004;58(4):1289–97.

40. Brunetti J, Caggiano A, Rosenbluth B, et al. Technical aspects of positron emission tomography/computed tomography fusion planning. Semin Nucl Med 2008;38(2):129–36.

41. Kidd EA, Siegel BA, Dehdashti F, et al. Clinical outcomes of definitive intensity-modulated radiation therapy with fluorodeoxyglucose-positron emission tomography simulation in patients with locally advanced cervical cancer. Int J Radiat Oncol Biol Phys 2010;77(4):1085–91.

42. Potter R, Dimopoulos J, Georg P, et al. Clinical impact of MRI assisted dose volume adaptation and dose escalation in brachytherapy of locally advanced cervix cancer. Radiother Oncol 2007;83:148–55.

43. Lin LL, Mutic S, Low DA, et al. Adaptive brachytherapy treatment planning for cervical cancer using FDG–PET. Int J Radiat Oncol Biol Phys 2007;67: 91–6.

44. Jacobs AJ, Faris C, Perez CA, et al. Short-term persistence of carcinoma of the uterine cervix after radiation: an indicator of long-term prognosis. Cancer 1986;57(5):944–50.

45. Hong JH, Tsai CS, Lai CH, et al. Recurrent squamous cell carcinoma of cervix after definitive radiotherapy. Int J Radiat Oncol Biol Phys 2004;60(1): 249–57.

46. Singh AK, Grigsby PW, Rader JS, et al. Cervix carcinoma, concurrent chemotherapy, and salvage of isolated paraaortic lymph node recurrence. Int J Radiat Oncol Biol Phys 2005;61(2):450–5.

47. Kong FM, Frey KA, Quint LE, et al. A pilot study of [18F]fluorodeoxyglucose positron emission tomography scans during and after radiation-based therapy in patients with non small cell lung cancer. J Clin Oncol 2007;25:3116–23.

48. Wieder HA, Brucher BL, Zimmermann F, et al. Time course of tumor metabolic activity during chemoradiation therapy of esophageal squamous cell carcinoma and response to treatment. J Clin Oncol 2004; 22:900–8.

49. Cascini GL, Avallone A, Delrio P, et al. 18F-FDG PET is an early predictor of pathologic tumor response to preoperative radiochemotherapy in locally advanced rectal cancer. J Nucl Med 2006;47:1241–8.

50. Grigsby PW, Siegel BA, Dehdashti F, et al. Post-therapy surveillance monitoring of cervical cancer by FDG-PET. Int J Radiat Oncol Biol Phys 2003;55: 907–13.

51. Grigsby PW, Siegel BA, Dehdashti F, et al. Post-therapy [18F] fluorodeoxyglucose positron emission tomography in carcinoma of the cervix: response and outcome. J Clin Oncol 2004;22:2167–71.

52. Schwarz JK, Siegel BA, Dehdashti F, et al. Association of posttherapy positron emission tomography with tumor response and survival in cervical carcinoma. JAMA 2007;298:2289–95.

53. Schwarz JK, Lin LL, Siegel BA, et al. 18-F-fluorodeoxyglucose-positron emission tomography evaluation of early metabolic response during radiation therapy for cervical cancer. Int J Radiat Oncol Biol Phys 2008;72(5):1502–7.

54. Kidd EA, Siegel BA, Dehdashti F, et al. The standardized uptake value for F-18 fluorodeoxyglucose is a sensitive predictive biomarker for cervical cancer treatment response and survival. Cancer 2007;110(8):1738–44.

55. Kidd EA, Grigsby PW. Intratumoral metabolic heterogeneity of cervical cancer. Clin Cancer Res 2008;14(16):5236–41.

56. Kidd EA. FDG-PET-based prognostic nomogram for locally advanced cervical cancer. American Radium Society 2010 Annual Meeting.

57. Bakkum-Gamez JN, Gonzalez-Bosquet J, Laack NN, et al. Current issues in the management of endometrial cancer. Mayo Clin Proc 2008;83(1):97–112.

58. Amant F, Moerman P, Neven P, et al. Endometrial cancer. Lancet 2005;366(9484):491–505.

59. Suzuki R, Miyagi E, Takahashi N, et al. Validity of positron emission tomography using fluoro-2-deoxyglucose for the preoperative evaluation of endometrial cancer. Int J Gynecol Cancer 2007; 17(4):890–6.

60. Picchio M, Mangili G, Samanes Gajate AM, et al. High-grade endometrial cancer: value of [(18)F] FDG PET/CT in preoperative staging. Nucl Med Commun 2010;31(6):506–12.

61. Park JY, Kim EN, Kim DY, et al. Comparison of the validity of magnetic resonance imaging and positron emission tomography/computed tomography in the preoperative evaluation of patients with uterine corpus cancer. Gynecol Oncol 2008;108(3):486–92.

62. Horowitz NS, Dehdashti F, Herzog TJ, et al. Prospective evaluation of FDG-PET for detecting pelvic and para-aortic lymph node metastasis in uterine corpus cancer. Gynecol Oncol 2004;95(3):546–51.

63. ASTEC study group, Kitchener H, Swart AM, Qian Q, et al. Efficacy of systematic pelvic lymphadenectomy in endometrial cancer (MRC ASTEC trial): a randomised study. Lancet 2009;373(9658):125–36.

64. Panici PB, Maggioni A, Hacker N, et al. Systematic aortic and pelvic lymphadenectomy versus resection of bulky nodes only in optimally debulked advanced ovarian cancer: a randomized clinical trial. J Natl Cancer Inst 2005;97(8):560–6.

65. Sugiyama T, Nishida T, Ushijima K, et al. Detection of lymph node metastasis in ovarian carcinoma and uterine corpus carcinoma by preoperative computerized tomography or magnetic resonance imaging. J Obstet Gynaecol (Tokyo 1995) 1995;21(6):551–6.

66. Rockall AG, Meroni R, Sohaib SA, et al. Evaluation of endometrial carcinoma on magnetic resonance imaging. Int J Gynecol Cancer 2007;17(1):188–96.

67. Rockall AG, Sohaib SA, Harisinghani MG, et al. Diagnostic performance of nanoparticle-enhanced magnetic resonance imaging in the diagnosis of lymph node metastases in patients with endometrial and cervical cancer. J Clin Oncol 2005;23(12): 2813–21.

68. Hricak H, Rubinstein LV, Gherman GM, et al. MR imaging evaluation of endometrial carcinoma: results of an NCI cooperative study. Radiology 1991;179(3):829–32.

69. Connor JP, Andrews JI, Anderson B, et al. Computed tomography in endometrial carcinoma. Obstet Gynecol 2000;95(5):692–6.

70. Manfredi R, Mirk P, Maresca G, et al. Local-regional staging of endometrial carcinoma: role of MR imaging in surgical planning. Radiology 2004;231(2):372–8.

71. Kitajima K, Nakamoto Y, Okizuka H, et al. Accuracy of 18F-FDG PET/CT in detecting pelvic and para-aortic lymph node metastasis in patients with endometrial cancer. AJR Am J Roentgenol 2008;190(6): 1652–8.

72. Lardinois D, Weder W, Hany TF, et al. Staging of non-small-cell lung cancer with integrated positron-emission tomography and computed tomography. N Engl J Med 2003;348(25):2500–7.

73. Sironi S, Buda A, Picchio M, et al. Lymph node metastasis in patients with clinical early-stage cervical cancer: detection with integrated FDG PET/CT. Radiology 2006;238(1):272–9.

74. Antoch G, Stattaus J, Nemat AT, et al. Non-small cell lung cancer: dual-modality PET/CT in preoperative staging. Radiology 2003;229(2):526–33.

75. Signorelli M, Guerra L, Buda A, et al. Role of the integrated FDG PET/CT in the surgical management of patients with high risk clinical early stage endometrial cancer: detection of pelvic nodal metastases. Gynecol Oncol 2009;115(2):231–5.

76. Bokhman JV. Two pathogenetic types of endometrial carcinoma. Gynecol Oncol 1983;15(1):10–7.

77. Nakamura K, Kodama J, Okumura Y, et al. The SUV-max of 18F-FDG PET correlates with histological grade in endometrial cancer. Int J Gynecol Cancer 2010;20(1):110–5.

78. Tsujikawa T, Yoshida Y, Mori T, et al. Uterine tumors: pathophysiologic imaging with 16 alpha-[F-18]fluoro-17 beta-estradiol and F-18 fluorodeoxyglucose PET-initial experience. Radiology 2008;248(2):599–605.

79. Tsujikawa T, Yoshida Y, Kudo T, et al. Functional images reflect aggressiveness of endometrial carcinoma: estrogen receptor expression combined with F-18-FDG PET. J Nucl Med 2009;50(10):1598–604.

Recent Advances in Hybrid Imaging for Radiation Therapy Planning: The Cutting Edge

Habib Zaidi, PhD, PD[a,b,*], Tinsu Pan, PhD[c]

KEYWORDS

- PET/CT • Radiation therapy • Treatment planning
- Respiratory motion • Image segmentation

PET/CT for radiation therapy planning (RTP) has been reported,[1–5] and it is expected that PET/CT will play an important role in the future of RTP or biologically guided radiation therapy (RT).[6,7] Integration of functional PET data with anatomic CT data should be a standard in RTP.[3] It remains a challenge, however, to quantify the improvement of simulation with PET/CT over CT in RTP because conclusive clinical data are not yet available. Early studies have found PET/CT has advantages over CT and MR imaging in the standardization of volume delineation,[8–11] in the reduction of the risk for geometric misses,[12] and in the minimization of radiation dose to the nontarget organs.[2,4,13] Utilization of PET/CT for RTP is expected to grow as more molecular targeted imaging agents are developed. Today, there are more than 2000 PubMed entries that result from a search using "PET" AND "Radiotherapy" (**Fig. 1**).

There are several challenges in PET/CT imaging for RTP. The first one is lack of reimbursement for PET/CT simulation. In the United States, each cancer patient is reimbursable for only one PET/CT scan before treatment, which may include surgery, chemotherapy, and radiation therapy (RT). This PET/CT scan is normally for diagnosis/staging. There are no data to support PET/CT simulation for NSCLC, esophageal, and head and neck patients, who are likely to benefit from PET/CT simulation. Most patients have their diseases characterized with the help of PET/CT before RT, and there is no reimbursement for PET/CT simulation for RT. This has significantly limited the application of PET/CT simulation for RT.

Patient setup and scan coverage are different between PET/CT imaging for diagnosis/staging and PET/CT imaging for RTP. The majority of PET/CT scans are performed in settings for disease diagnosis and patient management. It is typical to scan from the orbit to the midthigh for diagnosis/staging. The exception is head-to-toe coverage for melanoma cancer patients. The total time for scanning a patient is approximately 30 minutes, including patient setup time. Patient comfort and throughput are critical for the clinical operation. If PET/CT is used for RT, an immobilization device for the patient at treatment position should be made before fludeoxyglucose F 18 (^{18}F-FDG) injection to reduce the radiation exposure to the staff. After positioning the patient at the treatment

This work was supported by grant No. SNSF 31003A-125246 from the Swiss National Foundation and Geneva Cancer League.

[a] Division of Nuclear Medicine and Molecular Imaging, Geneva University Hospital, CH-1211 Geneva, Switzerland

[b] Geneva Neuroscience Center, Geneva University, CH-1211 Geneva, Switzerland

[c] Department of Imaging Physics, MD Anderson Cancer Center The University of Texas, Houston, TX 77030, USA

* Corresponding author. Division of Nuclear Medicine and Molecular Imaging, Geneva University Hospital, CH-1211 Geneva, Switzerland.

E-mail address: habib.zaidi@hcuge.ch

PET Clin 6 (2011) 207–226

doi:10.1016/j.cpet.2011.02.009

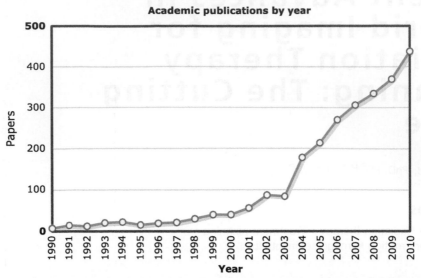

Fig. 1. The increasing number of annual peer-reviewed publications reporting on the use of PET and PET/CT in RT demonstrates the growing interest in PET-guided treatment planning. This graph is based on a PubMed query using the following MeSH terms: "RADIOTHERAPY" OR "RADIATION THERAPY" AND "POSITRON EMISSION TOMOGRAPHY". A timeline was created with MEDSUM, an online MEDLINE summary tool by MJ Galsworthy. Hosted by the Institute of Biomedical Informatics, Faculty of Medicine, University of Ljubljana, Slovenia (www. medsum.info.)

position, the disease area is scanned, such as the thorax for NSCLC and the head and the upper torso for head and neck cancer, unless the progression of the disease has changed after the diagnosis. Current PET/CT simulation procedures are mostly performed for the assessment of treatment response when RT is considered as a part of the treatment. If a limited coverage, such as the thorax or the head and neck area, can be prescribed for PET/CT simulation for RT, just like the current CT simulation for RT, the floodgate of PET/CT for RT will be opened. The continuing adoption of PET/CT to cover many disease indications and the continuing decline of reimbursement coupled with the drop of the PET/CT scanner are likely to open this floodgate in the future.

There are many factors that could affect the accuracy of quantification with PET/CT imaging for RT.[14] The most challenging one has been with imaging of the thoracic tumor or the NSCLC, in which respiratory motion could have an impact the diagnostic and staging accuracy. This review documents the recent technical advances in the field with special emphasis on the conceptual role of molecular PET/CT imaging RTP and the challenges arising from technical and physiologic factors that still need to be addressed. Much worthwhile research and development efforts remain to be done and many of the techniques reviewed are themselves not yet widely implemented in clinical settings.

NOVEL TRACERS AND TUMOR HYPOXIA

Recent advances in the development of novel tracers targeted to other aspects of tumor biology, including cell growth, cell death, oncogene expression, drug delivery, and tumor hypoxia, will significantly enhance the capability of clinical scientists to differentiate tumors and are likely to be used to guide treatment decisions. Several new tracers are expected to be approved and routinely used in the coming years.[15] The list of new tracers having the potential for routine use in the near future is long and not reviewed in this article. Interested readers may consult recently published reviews addressing this topic.[16–19] In certain cancers, ^{18}F-labeled fluorothymidine may prove to be of value in monitoring response to therapy instead of ^{18}F-FDG.[16] This tracer, however, does not seem optimal for diagnostic purposes because it is insensitive for detecting slow-growing tumors. ^{18}F-labeled DOPA[17] along with ^{68}Ga-labeled DOTA octreotide[18] and [124]I-metaiodobenzylguanidine[19] seem to have the promise of improving the management of patients with neuroendocrine tumors. Peptides containing amino acid sequence arginine-glycine-aspartate (RGD) seem to have an affinity toward integrins that are present on activated endothelial cells in tumors with angiogenesis.[20] ^{18}F-Galacto-RGD is a tracer developed for specific imaging of $\alpha_v\beta_3$ expression, a receptor involved in angiogenesis and metastasis that proved particularly useful in patients with squamous cell carcinoma of the head and neck.[21] Estrogen receptor targeting agents may be used to assess noninvasively the estrogen receptor section of tumors in vivo by ^{18}F-labeled estrogen analogues, such as fluoestradiol.[22] Angiogenesis, the formation of new vessels, is the target of a multitude of novel therapies and drugs. Therefore, direct visualization of this biologic response to tumor hypoxia and cell proliferation will be of great importance in developing these drugs. Peptides containing amino acid sequence RGD seem to have an affinity toward integrins that are present on activated endothelial cells in tumors with angiogenesis.[20] Apoptosis or programmed cell death can be imaged with radiolabeled Annex V to monitor response to therapy in cancer.[23]

Agents that measure regional hypoxia in malignant tumors (eg, FMISO, ^{18}F-EF5, and ^{64}Cu-ATSM) and possibly in some benign disorders will be frequently used,[24] especially in the context of RTP.[25] Tissue hypoxia is a pathologic condition in which a region of the body is deprived of adequate oxygen supply and is a major constraint for tumor treatment by RT. The efficacy of ionizing radiation directly relies on adequate supply of oxygen to the targeted tumor. As a tumor grows, it needs oxygen in order to survive. Although the tumor develops new blood vessels by a process of angiogenesis, these new vessels are typically less extensive than in normal tissues. As a result, the tumor cells do not receive adequate oxygen from the blood, leading to hypoxia and leaving portions of the tumor with regions where the oxygen concentration is significantly lower than in healthy tissues. Hypoxic tumor cells are usually resistant to RT and chemotherapy, but they can be made more susceptible to treatment by increasing the amount of oxygen in them. Furthermore, hypoxia is related to malignant progression, increased invasion, angiogenesis, and an increased risk of metastases formation.[26] There are three distinct types of tumor hypoxia[27]: (1) perfusion-related (acute) hypoxia, which results from inadequate blood flow in tumors; it is generally the consequence of recognized structural and functional abnormalities of the tumor neovasculature; (2) diffusion-related (chronic) hypoxia caused by increased oxygen diffusion distances due to tumor expansion; and (3) anemic hypoxia related to the reduced oxygen-carrying capacity of the blood.

Two different strategies can be used to overcome the problem of hypoxia-mediated radioresistance. The first strategy is to improve the tumor oxygenation during RT. The second strategy is to target hypoxia as a relatively unique feature of tumor tissue by means of drugs, which are activated under hypoxic conditions and act as hypoxic radiosensitizers or hypoxic cytotoxins.[26]

^{18}F-MISO and Cu-ATSM are the most widely used tracers in PET for their ability to demonstrate heterogeneity and general availability.[28] ^{18}F-MISO has relatively slow blood clearance and high lipophilicity contributing to significant background activity and relatively low contrast between hypoxic and normal tissues.[29] One remedy to this was to acquire a venous blood sample during the course of the imaging procedure for a tumor-to-blood ratio image to improve the contrast. ^{18}F-MISO is able to monitor the changing hypoxia status of lung tumors during RT.[30] Studies in sarcoma[31] and head and neck cancer[31,32] have demonstrated a correlation of ^{18}F-MISO uptake with poor outcome to radiation and chemotherapy.

Cu-ATSM is another promising agent for delineating the extent of hypoxia within tumors. Most Cu-ATSM studies have used the short-lived copper Cobalt-60 ([60]Cu) (half-life of 0.395 hours), which requires an on-site cyclotron. One advantage of using shorter-lived [60]Cu is the ability to perform multiple imaging sessions in a short time frame. To enable the transport of Cu-ATSM to the PET facilities without a cyclotron, longer-lived [61]Cu (half-life of 3.408 hours) and [64]Cu (half-life of 12.7 hours) are alternatives. Many preclinical studies have validated its use for imaging of hypoxia in tumors and other tissues. One concern with using Cu-ATSM to delineate hypoxia was that it may be tumor dependent, and cell-line dependent. It was demonstrated that there was variation in the ^{64}Cu-ATSM cellular accumulation, with uptake in normoxic cells being anywhere from 2 to 9 times lower than that in hypoxic cells, depending on the cell line. Nonetheless, ^{64}Cu-ATSM has been shown highly correlated with ^{18}F-FMISO in an animal model.[33] In human studies of lung[34] and cervical cancers,[35,36] [60]Cu-ATSM can act as a prognostic indicator for response to therapy. In a prospective study of 14 patients with NSCLC, a semiquantitative analysis of the [60]Cu-ATSM tumor-to-muscle ratio was able to discriminate those likely to respond to therapy from nonresponders.[37] A similar study in 14 women with cervical cancer demonstrated a similar predictive value in the tumor response to therapy. In the same study, tumor ^{18}F-FDG uptake did not correlate with [60]Cu-ATSM and there was no significant difference in tumor ^{18}F-FDG uptake between patients with hypoxic tumors and those with normoxic tumors.[37] ^{18}F-EF5 is another promising agent,[38,39] which proved useful for noninvasive clinical assessment of hypoxia in brain tumors.[40]

PET/CT-GUIDED RADIATION THERAPY

Early attempts to use nuclear medicine imaging, in particular PET, for RTP date back to the late 1990s.[41–48] An important contribution came from Ling and colleagues.[49] who established the concept of biologic imaging and moved forward the role of PET in RT, thus allowing it to enter the clinical arena. Since that time, the technical aspects of PET/CT-guided RT have been described more thoroughly in the scientific literature.[3,7,41–45,50–52] The success of these initial studies prompted significant interest from the major medical imaging equipment manufacturers, who all have introduced commercial PET/CT scanners equipped with the required accessories (flat couch insert, positioning system, respiratory gating, and other accessories) and software tools (virtual simulation, visualization and segmentation tools, support of Digital Imaging Communication in Medicine (DICOM) RT object definition, and other tools) for clinical use.[46] The typical workflow for PET/CT-guided RTP, usually involving two clinical departments (nuclear medicine and radiation oncology), is shown in **Fig. 2**.[7,47] With the growing

availability of large-bore dual-modality PET/CT scanners equipped with fixed RT positioning laser systems in the scanner room, a one-stop shop providing diagnostic PET/CT and RTP CT scan in only one session has become possible.[7]

The main motivation stimulating the use of PET/CT in RT is the efficacy of ^{18}F-FDG–PET imaging in a wide variety of malignant tumors with sensitivities, specificities, and accuracy often in the high 90th-percentile range.[48] In that sense, it might provide superior visualization compared with CT simulation, which in some cases might miss some areas that light up on the PET study, including the detection of distant metastases, or shed the light on the actual lesion volume, which might in reality be smaller on the PET study than on the CT alone. Moreover, discrepancies between anatomic (CT/MR imaging) and metabolic (PET) findings are often reported in the literature where the addition of PET has a significant impact on patient management and changed the treatment plans in 25% to 50% of cases.[1,3,5,53–61] Last and not least, interobserver and intraobserver variability was considerably reduced when PET information was available for target volume delineation.[8,62–65] Both state-of-the-art ^{18}F-FDG-PET and novel PET probes applications in the process of RTP are discussed elsewhere[7,66–68] and are beyond the scope of this review.

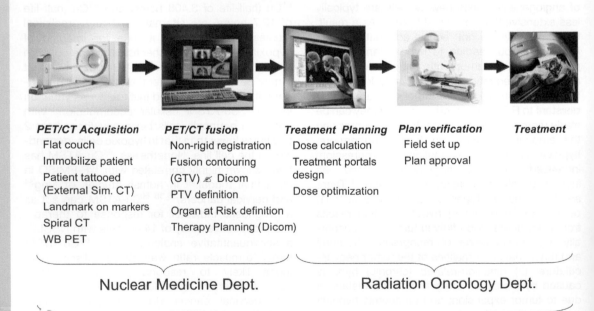

PET/CT Acquisition
Flat couch
Immobilize patient
Patient tattooed
(External Sim. CT)
Landmark on markers
Spiral CT
WB PET

PET/CT fusion
Non-rigid registration
Fusion contouring
(GTV) & Dicom
PTV definition
Organ at Risk definition
Therapy Planning (Dicom)

Treatment Planning
Dose calculation
Treatment portals design
Dose optimization

Plan verification
Field set up
Plan approval

Treatment

Nuclear Medicine Dept.   Radiation Oncology Dept.

Radiation Oncology Dept.

Fig. 2. Typical workflow for PET/CT-guided RTP where usually two clinical departments are involved (nuclear medicine and radiation oncology). Many academic radiation oncology facilities are now equipped with combined PET/CT scanners, which allows them to operate in complete autonomy.

Current indications for ^{18}F-FDG–PET/CT-guided RTP fall in two classes: established and experimental. Well-established indications include head and neck cancer, lung cancer, gynecologic cancer, and esophageal cancer whereas experimental indications comprise colorectal cancer, breast cancer, lymphoma and malignant melanoma, and many other malignancies.[7]

CHALLENGES OF PET/CT-GUIDED RADIATION THERAPY
Respiratory Motion

Misregistration between the CT and PET data due to the respiratory motion in the thorax and abdomen was reported soon after commercial PET/CT was introduced in 2001[53,69–72] and has been one of the most researched topics in PET/CT. Fast gantry rotation of less than 1 second per revolution and a large detector coverage of greater than 2 cm enable a CT scan of more than 100 cm in the cranial-caudal direction in 20 seconds. Alternatively, it normally takes 2 to 5 minutes to acquire the PET data of every 15 cm.[54,73] The temporal resolutions of CT and PET are different: less than 1 second for CT and approximately 1 respiratory cycle for PET. This mismatch in the temporal resolution may cause a misalignment of the tumor position between the CT and the PET data and may compromise quantification of the PET data.[66] The current design of PET/CT only matches the spatial resolutions of the CT and PET data by blurring the CT images so that the spatial resolution of the CT images matches the spatial resolution of the PET images. There has been no attempt from the manufacturers to match the temporal resolutions of CT and PET for a routine whole-body PET/CT scan.

Mismatch between the CT and PET data can be identified by a curvilinear white band or photopenic region at the diaphragm in the PET images. Existence of the white band only suggests a misregistration at the diaphragm. It is possible to have either a good registration or misregistration at the tumor location with or without a white band at the diaphragm. Because time is spent exhaling than inhaling, the PET data averaged over several minutes is closer to the end-exhale than the end-inhale. If the CT data are acquired near the end-exhale, then there is a good registration between the CT and the PET data. Alternatively, if the CT data are acquired in or near the end-inhale, the inflated lungs of inhale are larger than the deflated lungs of exhale. The larger area of the inflated lungs in CT renders less attenuation correction in the reconstruction of the PET data

near the diaphragm where the inflated lungs push the diaphragm lower in CT than the average diaphragm position in PET. The result is a white band region identified as the misregistered region or the photopenic region.

The rate of misregistration can be as high as 68%[67] to 84%.[70] It only has an impact on 2% of the diagnosis in a whole-body PET/CT with ^{18}F-FDG[74] and could be false positive in 40% of the cardiac PET/CT studies with Rubidium-82.[75] In the whole-body PET/CT for oncology, many lesions may not be close to the diaphragm where most misregistrations occur, and the task of diagnosis is generally not compromised by a misregistration between the CT and the PET data. Because the heart is right above the diaphragm, and the diagnosis of a cardiac PET is dependent on an accurate quantification of the PET data, a more stringent requirement in registration is needed for the cardiac PET/CT than for the whole-body PET/CT. For RT, a study of 216 patients in quantification with standardized uptake value (SUV) and gross target volume (GTV) delineation[67] indicated that 10% of the misregistrations could cause an SUV change of more than 25%, a threshold indicating a response to therapy,[76] and tumors of size less than 50 cm[3] near the diaphragm could have a change of the centroid tumor location of 2.4 mm, a GTV change of 154%, and an SUV change of 21%. More data are warranted to assess the impact of misregistration on RT.

Fast translation of the CT table during a helical CT scan may not eliminate or reduce misregistration between the CT and PET data. The CT images register better between slices if the CT scanner has at least 6 slices.[73] As long as the CT scan is conducted when the patient is free breathing, there are always some CT slices taken at inhale and some at exhale. The distance between the inhale and the exhale can become longer (or shorter) with a faster (or slower) speed helical CT scan. Fast CT gantry rotation can help freeze the motion and reduce motion artifacts in each CT slice and subsequently improves the PET image reconstruction. There is a difference between motion artifacts in each CT slice and registration of the CT images between slices. A fast gantry rotation speed can help reduce the motion artifacts in each CT slice. A faster helical CT scan with a higher pitch and a faster gantry rotation speed can help improve the registration between the CT slices. None of these can fix the problem of misregistration between the CT and PET data. **Fig. 3** shows an example of a whole-body helical CT scan in PET/CT with a 16-slice CT. There were respiratory artifacts on the abdomen and cardiac pulsation artifacts on the heart, which

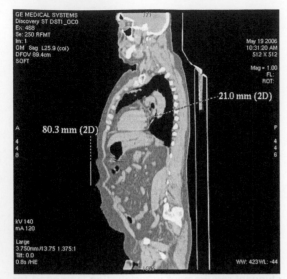

Fig. 3. An example of deriving the breathing cycle and heart rate from the motion artifacts in a free-breathing helical CT. There were breathing and cardiac pulsation artifacts on the abdomen and the heart in a free-breathing helical CT scan of pitch 1.375 to 1, x-ray collimation of 1 cm, and gantry rotation cycle of 0.8 second. The measured distances of periodicity were 80.3 mm and 21.0 mm for the breathing and cardiac pulsation artifacts, respectively. The speed of the helical CT scan was 17.2 m/s. The breathing cycle and the heart rate were estimated to be 4.67 seconds and 49 beats per minute.

were not discernible in the review of each individual CT slice. By measuring the distance between the adjacent peaks of the respiratory (cardiac pulsation) artifacts and dividing the distance to the table translation speed of the helical CT scan, the breathing cycle (the heat rate) of the patient can be estimated. These artifacts were due to the respiration and heart beating of the patient and are always with patient data. The presentation of the artifacts depends on the speed of the helical CT scan, however, and the breathing patterns of a patient during the helical CT scan.

Coaching patients to hold breath in the middle of exhale during the CT acquisition was suggested as a way to improve the registration of the CT and the PET data,[55] and the outcomes were mixed due to an unreliable coordination between patient and technologist. First, the definition of midexhale is subjective to patients. Breath hold at midexhale can mean midexhale in either a light or deep breathing. When a patient is asked to hold breath, there is a tendency for the patient to want to breathe in more air to maintain the subsequent midexhale breath hold. Second, a technologist has to give the breathing instruction and scan the patient at the same time, adding to the

complexity of operation. An example is shown in **Fig. 4.** More than 50% of the PET/CT data in a study of midexhale breath holds were with a white band at the diaphragm.[66] Today most clinics are scanning patients without any breathing instruction. In many cases, the registration between the CT and PET data for a patient in light breathing is often better than the one with coaching the patient to breath hold at the midexhale position.

One approach of improving the registration between the CT and the PET data is to bring the temporal resolution of the CT images to that of the PET data.[66] Because PET is averaged over many breath cycles, an average CT over 1 breath cycle helps improve the registration between the CT and the PET data. In this technique, the average CT data are acquired at a very high gantry rotation speed over 1 respiratory cycle. A scan of 4 seconds allows for 8 gantry rotations of 0.5 seconds. This is to ensure that each projection angle can collect as many phases of data as possible to allow data averaging over 1 respiratory cycle. Ideally, averaging the many projections or phases of the respiratory motion can be performed before image reconstruction. Current CT scanners do not have this function. Instead, multiple CT images of high temporal resolution are reconstructed and averaged for an average CT.[56] This is different from the slow CT scan technique with a slow gantry rotation of 4 seconds for an average CT, suggested by the American Association of Physicists in Medicine Task Group 76 for imaging the lung tumors not involved with either the mediastinum or the chest wall and not for the tumor of the liver, pancreas, and kidney.[57] A cine CT scan for average CT acquires consistent data in a fast CT rotation, and the object does not change its position much during a fast CT rotation. Alternatively, a slow scan CT acquires inconsistent data over a slow CT scan, producing the images with severe reconstruction artifacts due to the motion. A patient study is shown in **Fig. 5** to illustrate the difference in image quality between the average CT and slow scan CT at the diaphragm.

In terms of temporal resolution, average CT is similar to the transmission map acquired with 2 to 3 rotating transmission rod sources of Germanium-68 for attenuation correction of the PET data, shown to have an excellent registration with the emission PET data.[77,78] The advantages of cine CT averaging over transmission rod sources are (1) short acquisition time: 1 minute for cine CT and 10 minutes per 15 cm in transmission and (2) high photon flux and less noisy attenuation maps. The disadvantage is higher radiation dose (<0.83 mSv for the average CT acquired with

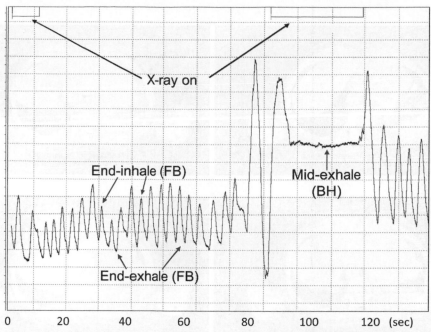

Fig. 4. A breathing trace of a patient during a helical CT scan. The two places of x-ray on are shown for the scout and helical CT scans. The patient was free breathing until a breathing instruction was given as "breath in, breath out," and hold your breath at midexhale. The difference between the breath-hold state and the free-breathing state caused a misalignment between the CT and the PET data. (*Reproduced from* Pan T, Mawlawi O, Nehmeh SA, et al. Attenuation correction of PET images with respiration-averaged CT images in PET/CT. J Nucl Med 2005;46:1481–87; with permission.)

10 mA for 5 s or 50 mAs and I<10 cm scanning) compared to approximately 0.13 mSv for the transmission rod sources.[79] Average CT can be sensitive to an irregular respiratory cycle during the data collection. One remedy for this is to acquire 2 respiratory cycles per table position so that an irregular respiratory cycle can be removed if needed. **Fig. 6** shows an example. By removing the irregularity, a normal average CT data can be obtained. RT has embraced the use of average CT for dose calculation,[58] in particular for proton beam therapy.[59] It has been shown that the average CT derived from cine CT is equivalent to the average CT from 4-D CT as far as dose calculation.[58] Because most of the new PET/CT scanners are not equipped with transmission rod sources, average CT cans serve as an alternative with the additional benefits in dose calculation for RT. **Fig. 7** shows an example of misregistration between the CT and the PET data and correction of misregistration by average CT to improve the accuracy of quantification for diagnosis. **Fig. 8** shows another example of misregistration that caused a false-negative diagnosis and a change of the location of the GTV for RT. In the era of image-guided RT, when RT can deliver a very high dose at great precision, it is important to

pay attention to any misregistration between the PET and the CT images during tumor delineation.

Average CT was first proposed for tumor imaging[66] and subsequently for cardiac imaging.[56] Its effectiveness was confirmed by other researchers[80,81] and in several clinical studies.[82–85] Although cine CT is associated with high radiation exposure for its long acquisition time, it should be applied judicially to the area of the targeted tumor with a radiation exposure of less than 5 mGy for diagnosis and less than 50 mGy for RT.[56] In comparison, the exposure of a typical diagnostic CT scan is approximately 20 mGy or higher. One way of minimizing the radiation dose is to apply average CT when there is a misregistration identified in the thorax or abdomen. In a typical PET/CT scan, the thorax and the abdomen images are available for review before the completion of the scan, and a decision to acquire average CT can be made accordingly. In RT, the amount of radiation is not a major concern due to the therapy dose of up to 70 Gy.

A novel technique to image patients at deep-inspiration breath hold (DIBH) for accurate quantification was first suggested by Nehmeh and colleagues[60] and has gained attention by several researchers.[61–65,68] Patients are asked to hold

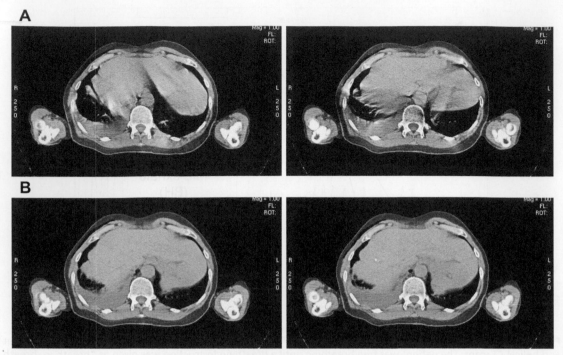

Fig. 5. The average CT (ACT) and the slow scan CT (SSCT) images of a patient with an average breath cycle of 4 seconds. The SSCT images (*A*) were taken with one single CT gantry rotation of 4 seconds, and the two images were taken with two separate acquisitions 2.5-mm apart and 2.5-mm thick. The corresponding ACT images (*B*), obtained by averaging the cine CT images, were averaged from 4 seconds of data collection over 8 gantry rotations. The ACT images were almost free of the reconstruction artifacts, evident in the SSCT images. (*Reproduced from* Pan T, Mawlawi O, Luo D, et al. Attenuation correction of PET cardiac data with low-dose average CT in PET/CT. Med Phys 2006;33:3931–8; with permission.)

breath at deep inspiration during CT and PET acquisition so that the tumor can be maintained stationary during the data acquisition. One study suggested a single DIBH of 20 seconds[63] and most studies used multiple DIBHs to improve the statistics of the PET data. There were some issues related to this technique: (1) applicability to the lung cancer patients with a compromised lung function, (2) potential mismatch between the CT and the PET data at DIBH, (3) reproducibility of the multiple DIBHs during the PET data acquisition, and (4) higher SUV due to the noisy PET data acquired in a duration of 1 or multiple breath holds. Some clinical data have suggested improvement in quantification and registration of the CT and the PET data with this technique. Because most of the RT procedures are conducted under normal breathing, this approach may be more applicable to staging and treatment response assessment than to RT simulation.

Respiratory gating is another important development in PET/CT for RT. In an evaluation of patients scanned in the past 6 years with a dedicated PET/CT scanner for RT in the University of Texas MD Anderson Cancer Center, Houston,

Texas, there were more than 4000 patients simulated with 4-D CT[77,86] and only 700 patients with PET/CT. In terms of demographics, all thoracic RT patients for lung, esophageal, or liver disease were 4-D CT simulated. Iodinated contrast media was incorporated in 4-D CT imaging of the liver tumor to enhance the contrast between the liver tumor and the parenchyma for treatment planning.[74] For the 700 PET/CT scans, there were 63% for non–small cell lung cancer (NSCLC), 14% for esophageal cancer, 13% for head and neck cancer, 1% for solitary pulmonary nodules, and 9% for the other indications. The PET/CT scans for RT were performed when staging was requested and RT was included in the treatment. The number of PET/CT scans performed on this scanner was limited because there was only one PET/CT scan reimbursed per patient before treatment, and the PET/CT scan is normally conducted for the purpose of diagnosis, not for RT. In total, there were 64% of the 700 PET/CT scans (NSCLC and solitary pulmonary nodules) of lung cancer. This is in contrast to an average of 32% PET/CT procedures performed for the lung cancer in general.[87] If the esophageal cancer patients are

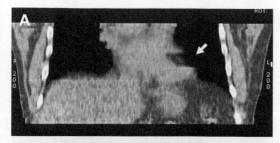

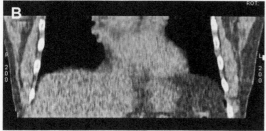

Fig. 6. (A) The average CT image from a cine acquisition of 10 seconds, which is approximately 2 respiratory cycles, and (B) the average CT image from 5 seconds or 50% of the 10-second cine CT data after removing an irregular respiratory cycle of data pointed by an arrow (A). This example demonstrated the importance of regular respiration in the cine CT acquisition and the potential of removing an irregularity to derive a normal average CT if there is more than 1 respiratory cycle of data to choose from.

included, there were almost 78% of the RT PET/CT patients for whom the tumor motion from respiration was assessed with 4-D CT in a single session of PET/CT simulation. The PET data were attenuation corrected with average CT from the cine CT data in 4-D CT to improve the registration of the CT and the PET data.

Although 4-D PET[88] can also be performed on this PET/CT for RT, its application has been limited due to the total acquisition time approaching 40 minutes.[89] Most patients cannot hold their arms up over their heads for more than 30 minutes and the long acquisition time could induce patient motion and compromise the PET/CT study. Moreover, the statistics of 4-D PET is poor due to splitting up the coincidence events into multiple bins or phases for 4-D PET, and the spatial resolution of PET in general is only approximately 5 to 10 mm.[90] In a recent clinical investigation of 18 patients with 4-D PET,[89] it was found that respiratory gating increases SUV by 22.4% and improves the consistency of tumor volumes between PET and CT. This study was the first clinical investigation reported since the introduction of 4-D PET/CT in 2004.[91] In contrast, 4-D CT can be performed in less than 2 minutes for the coverage of the whole lungs. There is normally high contrast

between the lung tumor and the parenchyma except when the lung tumor is connected to a similar tissue density of the mediastinum and chest wall. It is relatively easy to incorporate 4-D CT than 4-D PET in a PET/CT simulation.

List-mode data acquisition,[92] extension of axial field of view,[93] and time-of-flight[82] technologies could in the future catapult 4-D PET into a routine clinical procedure. Today many PET/CT scanners can acquire the list-mode PET data to reconstruct a static PET data set as in a routine PET scan. The same list-mode data can also be reconstructed for the gated PET data if the corresponding respiratory signal were recorded during data acquisition. The advantage of this approach is that the static data can be used as a part of the gated data to offset the long acquisition time for 4-D PET. Increasing the axial field of view from 15 to 22 cm can increase the sensitivity of data acquisition and shorten the scan time of 4-D PET. The time-of-flight technology, which helps localize more accurately each coincidence event in the image space than the conventional PET without time of flight, can improve the signal-to-noise ratio and reduce the scan time of 4-D PET.[82] Integration of the new technologies in a clinic environment with an efficient image reconstruction process and a simple workflow are critical for 4-D PET to be clinically feasible.

Partial Volume Effect

Partial volume effect (PVE) is the underestimation of activity concentration in a lesion due to the limited spatial resolution of PET, which is in the range of 5 to 10 mm for clinical PET/CT systems. PVE has an impact on most quantification of small lesions of size less than 2 to 3 times the PET spatial resolution.[83,94] Any factor contributing to image reconstruction, image filtering, and presentation of images also has an impact on PVE. It is also related to the metric used to measure the activity concentration, such as the maximum activity concentration of a voxel or the average activity concentration of a volume in a tumor. The most used metric is the maximum SUV, which is sensitive to the noise but not dependent on the selection of a volume as is in the average activity concentration. In general, a tumor of size less than 3 cm look larger but less aggressive than it actually is in PET.[83,94] Although it has been 30 years since PVE was researched and attempted for correction,[95] correction of PVE in PET imaging is not yet clinically available.

Several approaches have been proposed to compensate for the PVE[83] with many of them developed specifically for brain imaging.[94] These can

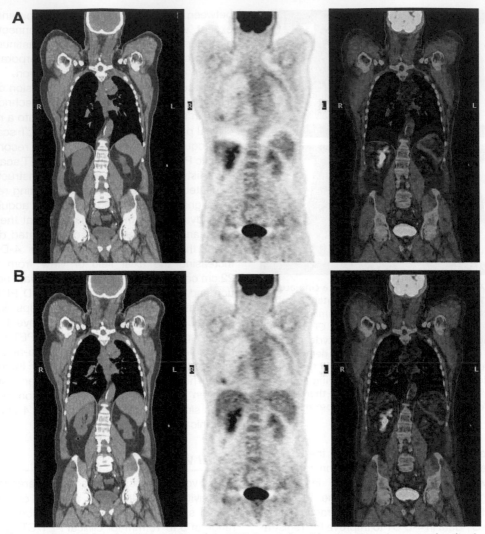

Fig. 7. The CT, PET, and fused PET/CT images of an NSCLC patient with misregistration near the diaphragm are shown (*A*), and the corresponding images with attenuation correction with the average CT data are shown (*B*). The maximum SUV increased 57% from 2.3 (*A*) to 3.6 (*B*). In this comparison, the same PET data were reconstructed with the conventional CT (*A*) and average CT (*B*).

broadly be divided into (1) postreconstruction-based methods and (2) reconstruction-based methods. Each of these two categories can be implemented in the form of either region of interest (ROI)-based or voxel-based approaches. Potential advantages of PVE-corrected images, as opposed to PVE-corrected ROI-measured concentrations, include the capability to accurately outline functional volumes as well as improving tumor-to-background ratio, which could considerably improve diagnostic examinations, studies involving the assessment of response to treatment, and PET-based RTP. In this context, however, the problem is more complex and relies in many cases on a number of often-strong assumptions and approximations.[94]

Recovery coefficient (RC) is a simple method of estimating the true quantitative value if the tumor of interest has a size and shape similar to the ones already modeled through simulation or measurement.[95] It can be implemented with a look-up table and can be computationally efficient. For a spherical tumor, the RC can be derived as a function of the sphere size and the signal-to-background ratio (SBR) for a wide range of spatial resolution values.[96] A simple correction can be performed by dividing the measured activity with the RC corresponding to the size and shape of the metabolically active tumor. Homogeneous activity concentration and simple geometry tumors are easier for the correction with RC than the inhomogeneous activity concentration and

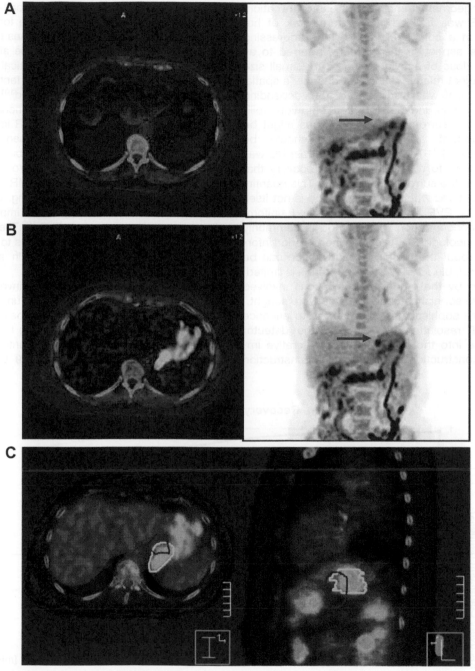

Fig. 8. The PET/CT images of a 69-year-old female patient with an esophageal tumor after induction chemo-therapy. (A) Shows an axial slice of the fused clinical CT and PET image at the level of the esophageal tumor (*left*) and the PET image in coronal view (*right*). The radiology report indicated the patient had a positive response to the chemotherapy. After removal of misalignment by the average CT, the tumor reappeared in the same PET data set (B). The arrows point to the tumor location. The GTVs drawn in the images (A) and (B) are shown in blue and in green, respectively (C). The patient was treated with the tumor volume in green, and the radiology report was corrected by the average CT. (*Reproduced from* Pan T, Mawlawi O. PET/CT in radiation oncology. Med Phys 2008;35:4955–66; with permission.)

irregular geometry tumors. In this early publication, the PVE was tackled in the framework of hot objects in a cold background, thus addressing only one aspect of the problem, referred to as spill-out (loss of activity owing to the small size of the object relative to the PET scanner's spatial resolution). It was also realized that, depending on the background's activity concentration, spill-in from the surrounding warm tissues might be as important as spill-out and should be compensated.[94] The concept of contrast RC was introduced[96] to reflect the rate of recovery that lies above the surrounding medium. This quantity is only justified when the background is not itself subject to PVE and is of known and uniform activity concentration. The method is commonly used in oncologic PET imaging where a priori information about the tumor size and shape can be made available.[78–80,97–99] The approach is limited, however, by the crude approximations involved and more sophisticated techniques were sought.

A more sophisticated approach is to enhance the PET resolution by modeling the detector response into the system matrix in iterative image reconstruction[81,84] because reconstruction methods that improve the effective spatial resolution of the scanner can compensate for PVE. In this sense, there are many approaches to reconstruction that attempt to achieve the aforementioned goals[85,100]; the use of statistical iterative reconstructions has been an important step in this direction both for voxel-based[101,102] and ROI-based[103–106] reconstructions. Incorporation of the anatomic information from MR imaging in the reconstruction has been proposed for brain imaging[107] and might in the future be extended to other applications with the introduction of dual-modality whole-body PET/MR imaging systems.[108] Deconvolution, deblurring, or image restoration can also be applied to improve the image resolution and reduce PVE.[109] The computation load of these approaches tends to be large and may hinder their application in a clinical setting.

Because PET/CT for RT is typically involved with lung cancer and esophageal cancer, tumor motion is another component complicating the correction of PVE. It is difficult if not impossible to separate tumor motion from PVE as far as quantification of the PET data is concerned. **Fig. 9** shows an

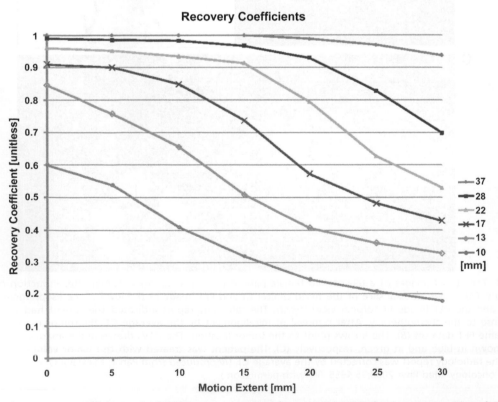

Fig. 9. The recovery coefficients of a PET/CT system measured from a NEMA IEC phantom on a motion platform. There were 6 spheres of size, 10, 13, 17, 22, 28, and 37 mm, and 7 motion amplitudes of 0 to 30 mm in increments of 5 mm. The SBR was 50:1. Each data point was averaged from 3 measurements.

example of RC as a function of different sphere sizes (10, 13, 17, 22, 28, and 37 mm) and various degrees of motion (no motion to 30 mm) by measuring the degradation of a known activity with the image quality phantom IEC phantom at the SBR of 50:1. Tumor motion adds another dimension of degradation on top of the PVE. Incorporation of 4-D CT to help assess the magnitude of tumor motion and the size and shape of the tumor from CT can be helpful in modeling both the tumor motion and system resolution in image reconstruction[110] or image deconvolution[88,111] to simultaneously compensate for both motion and PVE. One such approach applied successfully in the context of oncologic PET imaging uses an iterative 3-D deconvolution algorithm and a local model of the PET scanner's point spread function followed by application of a PVE correction to the mean voxel value within a VOI.[109] The authors report more accurate quantitative assessments of uptake in lesions greater than 1.5 times the PET imaging spatial resolution.

A different, novel type of approach to this problem has been to directly quantify ROIs from projection data, taking the effect of PVE (among others factors such as scatter) into account. Derived from the early work of Huesman,[103] this approach has been developed and investigated in the context of oncologic imaging.[91,112] This method has the particular advantage of being able to estimate region variance for subsequent use in model analysis to obtain parameter estimates; however, this method remains to be extended to 3-D.

PET Image Segmentation

Over the past few years, several methods have been proposed for target volume definition in RTP based on incorporating PET physiologic information. In particular, ^{18}F-FDG-PET is currently used in many cancer centers around the world to improve biologic target volume definition, which is traditionally identified on CT simulation images in RT clinical routine.[113] Accurate volume definition is particularly important in RT because it constitutes the target of the radiation beam; underdosing of tumor may lead to recurrence whereas overdosing of surrounding normal tissues might lead to severe and possibly lethal side effects to patients, such as brain or lung injury.[114] Different approaches can be followed to categorize PET segmentation approaches, including the cancer site, the injected radiotracer, or the image processing technique. There could be differences and overlaps between sites, tracers, or techniques. For many reasons, the authors

have opted to categorize PET segmentation based on the techniques used and refer to differences in sites or tracer specific variations as appropriate.[115] There is a plethora of segmentation methods that could be applied to nuclear medicine imaging, particularly in cardiovascular imaging; readers are referred to articles by Boudrass and colleageus.[116,117] According to a literature survey of existing methods, the authors identified 4 broad categories of PET segmentation methodologies: (1) image thresholding methods, (2) variational approaches, (3) learning methods, and (4) stochastic modeling-based techniques.[46] A detailed description of these algorithms is beyond the scope of this review and can be found in that survey.

Thresholding is the most widely used PET segmentation approach in clinical practice for biologic target volume delineation for RTP. The only competing approach with thresholding is possibly visual interpretation of PET scans and identification of lesion boundary by consensus reading of an experienced nuclear medicine physician and radiation oncologist.[118,119] Visual inspection is susceptible to the window-level settings, however, and suffers from interobserver variability. Therefore, several segmentation methods based on thresholding have emerged to reduce this subjectivity. There is a large variability in terms of computational complexity and amount of user interaction required by the various image segmentation techniques. Despite their limitations, visual delineation performed by experts is still the most widely used technique.[8] Manual techniques, however, are labor intensive and suffer from intraobserver variability whereas thresholding techniques are simple to put into practice, although scanner-specific calibration might be required for implementation of the adaptive thresholding method. The high computational burden associated with supervised methods that require time-consuming training is also worth emphasizing. In a clinical setting, the balance between algorithmic complexity and the validity of results obtained is an important criterion when selecting a PET image segmentation technique.

A challenging, even problematic, issue for validation of PET segmentation algorithms, is the identification of a gold standard (ie, benchmark).[120,121] Segmentation methods yield binary classification results (a voxel belongs to the object or does not). There are basically 4 different strategies allowing the assessment of the accuracy of PET image segmentation techniques. The review by Zaidi and El Naqa[46] summarizes these strategies and provides a concise summary of their advantages, drawbacks and limitations. These include manual segmentation by experts in the field, the use of simulated or experimental phantom studies where the ground truth (tumor volume) is known a priori, the comparison with correlated anatomic GTVs defined on CT or MR imaging, and the comparison of tumor volumes delineated on clinical PET data with actual tumor volumes measured on the macroscopic specimen derived from histology, in case a PET scan was undertaken before surgery. It should be emphasized that such correlative analysis relies on a high degree of registration accuracy between multimodality images, which is still challenging to perform in a clinical setting.[122]

Many studies compared various PET image segmentation techniques using phantom and clinical studies. For example, Vees and colleagues[11] compared various image segmentation techniques in the delineation of GTV in patients with cerebral glioma (**Fig. 10**). The study results highlighted the limitations associated with some of

the segmentation algorithms (eg, SUV = 2.5 cutoff and the gradient finding GTV approaches) compared with the SBR-based adaptive thresholding technique and its impact on RT planning in patients of cerebral glioma. The investigators concluded the selection of the most appropriate ^{18}F-FET-PET–based segmentation algorithm is crucial for correct delineation of resulting GTV.[11]

A recent study compared 9 PET image segmentation techniques.[123] These include manual delineation performed by an experienced radiation oncologist on both the CT and PET images, 4 semi-automated methods comprising the SBR-based adaptive thresholding technique,[124] region growing,[125] Black and colleagues' technique,[126] Nestle and colleagues' technique,[127] and 3 fully automated methods: standard fuzzy C-means[128]; spatial FCM, which incorporates nonlinear anisotropic diffusion filtering, thus allowing the integration of spatial contextual information; and the wavelet-based FCM-S algorithm, which also

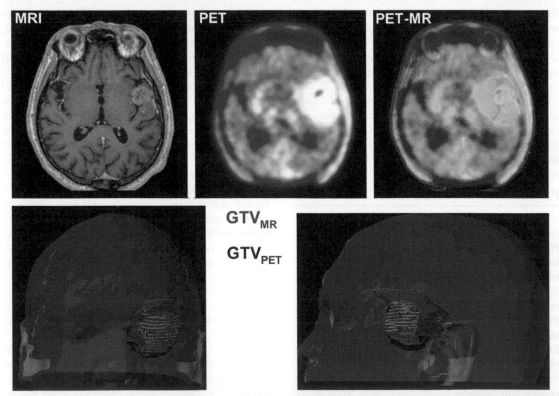

Fig. 10. Typical example of geographic mismatch between GTVs defined on MR imaging and PET for a clinical study with a glioblastoma. (*Top*) From left to right, gadolinium-enhanced T1-weighted MR imaging, corresponding ^{18}F-FET–PET study, and fused PET/MR imaging. (*Bottom*) 3-D rendering illustrating the substantial mismatch. Note that the GTV defined on MR imaging overestimates the tumor extension relative to GTV defined on PET images. (*Adapted from* Weber DC, Zilli T, Buchegger F, et al. [(18)F]fluoroethyltyrosine-positron emission tomography-guided radiotherapy for high-grade glioma. Radiat Oncol 2008;3:44; with permission; and Vees H, Senthamizhchelvan S, Miralbell R, et al. Assessment of various strategies for 18F-FET PET-guided delineation of target volumes in high-grade glioma patients. Eur J Nucl Med Mol Imaging 2009;36:182–93; with permission.)

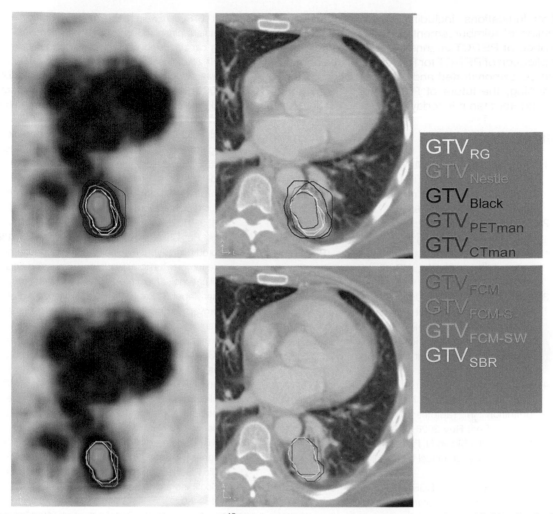

Fig. 11. Representative segmentation results of ^{18}F-FDG-PET/CT image of a patient presenting with histologically proved NSCLC. The gross tumor volumes defined on the ellipsoidal homogeneous lesion using 9 segmentation techniques are depicted on both the CT (*left*) and ^{18}F-FDG-PET (*right*) transaxial slices.

considers inhomogeneity of tracer uptake through the use of the à trou wavelet transform.[129] Representative segmentation results of ^{18}F-FDG-PET/CT image of a patient presenting with histologically proved NSCLC are shown in **Fig. 11**. The GTVs defined on the nonhomogeneous lesion using 9 segmentation techniques are depicted on both the CT (left) and ^{18}F-FDG-PET (right) transaxial slices.

SUMMARY AND FUTURE PERSPECTIVES

There have been many contributions demonstrating the advantages of combining morphologic and molecular imaging in the process of RTP thanks to the widespread acceptance of combined PET/CT scanners. The emergence of novel technologies, including PET/MR imaging,

will likely boost further the application of multimodality imaging in RT for various indications. Molecular imaging-guided RT holds the promise of improved delineation of tumor target volumes. Yet, despite considerable progress to date, challenges remain if the potential of PET/CT-guided RTP is to be fully exploited in clinical routine.

PET/CT has been mainly used for whole-body oncologic studies, an application embracing the mainstream of reimbursable indications for PET/CT in the United States and many other countries. Reimbursement issues are mainly driven by prospective multicenter clinical trials that reveal enhancements in health outcomes conveyed by PET/CT as an imaging modality for a given indication. It is expected that ongoing collaborative efforts will allow expanding coverage for PET/CT scans by following the same trend adopted for other indications, including RTP. The continuing decline of reimbursement coupled with the drop in price of PET/CT scanners are likely to help the application of PET/CT for RT. After all, if the benefit can be demonstrated and if the cost of scans are dropping, the future of PET/CT for RT can only be brighter than it is today.

REFERENCES

1. Bradley J, Thorstad WL, Mutic S, et al. Impact of FDG-PET on radiation therapy volume delineation in non-small-cell lung cancer. Int J Radiat Oncol Biol Phys 2004;59:78–86.

2. Ciernik IF, Dizendorf E, Baumert BG, et al. Radiation treatment planning with an integrated positron emission and computer tomography (PET/CT): a feasibility study. Int J Radiat Oncol Biol Phys 2003;57:853–63.

3. Mah K, Caldwell CB, Ung YC, et al. The impact of (18)FDG-PET on target and critical organs in CT-based treatment planning of patients with poorly defined non-small-cell lung carcinoma: a prospective study. Int J Radiat Oncol Biol Phys 2002;52:339–50.

4. van Baardwijk A, Baumert BG, Bosmans G, et al. The current status of FDG-PET in tumor volume definition in radiotherapy treatment planning. Cancer Treat Rev 2006;32:245–60.

5. Messa C, Di Muzio N, Picchio M, et al. PET/CT and radiotherapy. Q J Nucl Med Mol Imaging 2006;50:4–14.

6. Stewart RD, Li XA. BGRT: biologically guided radiation therapy—the future is fast approaching. Med Phys 2007;34:3739–51.

7. Zaidi H, Vees H, Wissmeyer M. Molecular PET/CT imaging-guided radiation therapy treatment planning. Acad Radiol 2009;16:1108–33.

8. Steenbakkers RJ, Duppen JC, Fitton I, et al. Reduction of observer variation using matched CT-PET for lung cancer delineation: a three-dimensional analysis. Int J Radiat Oncol Biol Phys 2006;64:435–48.

9. Ashamalla H, Rafla S, Parikh K, et al. The contribution of integrated PET/CT to the evolving definition of treatment volumes in radiation treatment planning in lung cancer. Int J Radiat Oncol Biol Phys 2005;63:1016–23.

10. Weber DC, Zilli T, Buchegger F, et al. [(18)F]Fluoroethyltyrosine-positron emission tomography-guided radiotherapy for high-grade glioma. Radiat Oncol 2008;3:44.

11. Vees H, Senthamizhchelvan S, Miralbell R, et al. Assessment of various strategies for 18F-FET PET-guided delineation of target volumes in high-grade glioma patients. Eur J Nucl Med Mol Imaging 2009;36:182–93.

12. Erdi YE, Rosenzweig K, Erdi AK, et al. Radiotherapy treatment planning for patients with non-small cell lung cancer using positron emission tomography (PET). Radiother Oncol 2002;62:51–60.

13. Schwartz DL, Ford EC, Rajendran J, et al. FDG-PET/CT-guided intensity modulated head and neck radiotherapy: a pilot investigation. Head Neck 2005;27:478–87.

14. Zaidi H. Quantitative analysis in nuclear medicine imaging. In: Zaidi H, editor. New York: Springer; 2006. p. 564.

15. Zaidi H, Alavi A. Preface. PET Clin 2007;2:xi–xiv.

16. Mankoff D, Shields A, Krohn K. PET imaging of cellular proliferation. Radiol Clin North Am 2005;43:153–67.

17. Jager PL, Chirakal R, Marriott CJ, et al. 6-L-18F-Fluorodihydroxyphenylalanine PET in neuroendocrine tumors: basic aspects and emerging clinical applications. J Nucl Med 2008;49:573–86.

18. Milker-Zabel S, Zabel-du Bois A, Henze M, et al. Improved target volume definition for fractionated stereotactic radiotherapy in patients with intracranial meningiomas by correlation of CT, MRI, and [68Ga]-DOTATOC-PET. Int J Radiat Oncol Biol Phys 2006;65:222–7.

19. Shapiro B. Ten years of experience with MIBG applications and the potential of new radiolabeled peptides: a personal overview and concluding remarks. Q J Nucl Med 1995;39:150–5.

20. Belvisi L, Bernardi A, Colombo M, et al. Targeting integrins: insights into structure and activity of cyclic RGD pentapeptide mimics containing azabicycloalkane amino acids. Bioorg Med Chem 2006;14:169–80.

21. Beer AJ, Grosu AL, Carlsen J, et al. [18F]Galacto-RGD positron emission tomography for imaging of {alpha}v{beta}3 expression on the neovasculature in patients with squamous cell carcinoma of the head and neck. Clin Cancer Res 2007;13:6610–6.

22. Couturier O, Luxen A, Chatal JF, et al. Fluorinated tracers for imaging cancer with positron emission tomography. Eur J Nucl Med Mol Imaging 2004;31:1182–206.

23. Blankenberg F, Katsikis P, Tait J, et al. In vivo detection and imaging of phosphatidylserine expression during programmed cell death. Proc Natl Acad Sci U S A 1998;95:6349–54.

24. Rajendran J, Krohn K. Imaging hypoxia and angiogenesis in tumors. Radiol Clin North Am 2005;43:169–87.

25. Thorwarth D, Alber M. Implementation of hypoxia imaging into treatment planning and delivery. Radiother Oncol 2010;97:172–5.

26. Weinmann M, Welz S, Bamberg M. Hypoxic radiosensitizers and hypoxic cytotoxins in radiation oncology. Curr Med Chem Anticancer Agents 2003;3:364–74.

27. Vaupel P, Harrison L. Tumor hypoxia: causative factors, compensatory mechanisms, and cellular response. Oncologist 2004;9(Suppl 5):4–9.

28. Padhani A. PET imaging of tumor hypoxia. Cancer Imaging 2006;6:S117–21.

29. Nunn A, Linder K, Strauss HW. Nitroimidazoles and imaging hypoxia. Eur J Nucl Med 1995;22:265–80.

30. Koh WJ, Bergman KS, Rasey JS, et al. Evaluation of oxygenation status during fractionated radiotherapy in human nonsmall cell lung cancers using [F-18]fluoromisonidazole positron emission tomography. Int J Radiat Oncol Biol Phys 1995;33:391–8.

31. Rajendran JG, Wilson DC, Conrad EU, et al. [(18)F]FMISO and [(18)F]FDG PET imaging in soft tissue sarcomas: correlation of hypoxia, metabolism and VEGF expression. Eur J Nucl Med Mol Imaging 2003;30:695–704.

32. Hicks RJ, Rischin D, Fisher R, et al. Utility of FMISO PET in advanced head and neck cancer treated with chemoradiation incorporating a hypoxia-targeting chemotherapy agent. Eur J Nucl Med Mol Imaging 2005;32:1384–91.

33. Dence CS, Ponde DE, Welch MJ, et al. Autoradiographic and small-animal PET comparisons between (18)F-FMISO, (18)F-FDG, (18)F-FLT and the hypoxic selective (64)Cu-ATSM in a rodent model of cancer. Nucl Med Biol 2008;35:713–20.

34. Dehdashti F, Mintun MA, Lewis JS, et al. In vivo assessment of tumor hypoxia in lung cancer with 60Cu-ATSM. Eur J Nucl Med Mol Imaging 2003; 30:844–50.

35. Grigsby PW, Malyapa RS, Higashikubo R, et al. Comparison of molecular markers of hypoxia and imaging with (60)Cu-ATSM in cancer of the uterine cervix. Mol Imaging Biol 2007;9:278–83.

36. Dehdashti F, Grigsby PW, Lewis JS, et al. Assessing tumor hypoxia in cervical cancer by PET with 60Cu-labeled diacetyl-bis(N4-methylthiosemicarbazone). J Nucl Med 2008;49:201–5.

37. Dehdashti F, Grigsby PW, Mintun MA, et al. Assessing tumor hypoxia in cervical cancer by positron emission tomography with 60Cu-ATSM: relationship to therapeutic response-a preliminary report. Int J Radiat Oncol Biol Phys 2003;55:1233–8.

38. Dolbier WR Jr, Li AR, Koch CJ, et al. [18F]-EF5, a marker for PET detection of hypoxia: synthesis of precursor and a new fluorination procedure. Appl Radiat Isot 2001;54:73–80.

39. Komar G, Seppanen M, Eskola O, et al. 18F-EF5: a new PET tracer for imaging hypoxia in head and neck cancer. J Nucl Med 2008;49:1944–51.

40. Evans S, Hahn S, Judy K, et al. 18F EF5 PET imaging with imunohistochemical validation in patients with brain lesions [abstract]. Int J Radiat Oncol Biol Phys 2006;66:S248.

41. Yap JT, Carney JP, Hall NC, et al. Image-guided cancer therapy using PET/CT. Cancer J 2004;10:221–33.

42. Bradley JD, Perez CA, Dehdashti F, et al. Implementing biologic target volumes in radiation treatment planning for non-small cell lung cancer. J Nucl Med 2004;45(Suppl 1):96S–101S.

43. Brunetti J, Caggiano A, Rosenbluth B, et al. Technical aspects of positron emission tomography/computed tomography fusion planning. Semin Nucl Med 2008;38:129–36.

44. Pan T, Mawlawi O. PET/CT in radiation oncology. Med Phys 2008;35:4955–66.

45. Nestle U, Weber W, Hentschel M, et al. Biological imaging in radiation therapy: role of positron emission tomography. Phys Med Biol 2009;54:R1–25.

46. Zaidi H, El Naqa I. PET-guided delineation of radiation therapy treatment volumes: a survey of image segmentation techniques. Eur J Nucl Med Mol Imaging 2010;37:2165–87.

47. Macapinlac HA. Clinical applications of positron emission tomography/computed tomography treatment planning. Semin Nucl Med 2008;38:137–40.

48. Czernin J, Allen-Auerbach M, Schelbert HR. Improvements in cancer staging with PET/CT: Literature-based evidence as of september 2006. J Nucl Med 2007;48:78S–88S.

49. Ling CC, Humm J, Larson S, et al. Towards multidimensional radiotherapy (MD-CRT): biological imaging and biological conformality. Int J Radiat Oncol Biol Phys 2000;47:551–60.

50. Chapman JD, Bradley JD, Eary JF, et al. Molecular (functional) imaging for radiotherapy applications: an RTOG symposium. Int J Radiat Oncol Biol Phys 2003;55:294–301.

51. Paulino AC, Thorstad WL, Fox T. Role of fusion in radiotherapy treatment planning. Semin Nucl Med 2003;33:238–43.

52. Scarfone C, Lavely WC, Cmelak AJ, et al. Prospective feasibility trial of radiotherapy target definition for head and neck cancer using 3-dimensional PET and CT imaging. J Nucl Med 2004; 45:543–52.

53. Osman MM, Cohade C, Nakamoto Y, et al. Clinically significant inaccurate localization of lesions with PET/CT: frequency in 300 patients. J Nucl Med 2003;44:240–3.

54. Beyer T, Antoch G, Muller S, et al. Acquisition protocol considerations for combined PET/CT imaging. J Nucl Med 2004;45(Suppl 1):25S–35S.

55. Goerres GW, Burger C, Schwitter MR, et al. PET/CT of the abdomen: optimizing the patient breathing pattern. Eur Radiol 2003;13:734–9.

56. Pan T, Mawlawi O, Luo D, et al. Attenuation correction of PET cardiac data with low-dose average CT in PET/CT. Med Phys 2006;33:3931–8.

57. Keall PJ, Mageras GS, Balter JM, et al. The management of respiratory motion in radiation oncology report of AAPM Task Group 76. Med Phys 2006; 33:3874–900.

58. Riegel AC, Ahmad M, Sun X, et al. Dose calculation with respiration-averaged CT processed from cine CT without a respiratory surrogate. Med Phys 2008; 35:5738–47.

59. Cai J, Read PW, Baisden JM, et al. Estimation of error in maximal intensity projection-based internal target volume of lung tumors: a simulation and comparison study using dynamic magnetic resonance imaging. Int J Radiat Oncol Biol Phys 2007;69:895–902.

60. Nehmeh SA, Erdi YE, Meirelles GS, et al. Deep-inspiration breath-hold PET/CT of the thorax. J Nucl Med 2007;48:22–6.

61. Nagamachi S, Wakamatsu H, Kiyohara S, et al. The reproducibility of deep-inspiration breath-hold (18) F-FDG PET/CT technique in diagnosing various cancers affected by respiratory motion. Ann Nucl Med 2010;24:171–8.

62. Daisaki H, Shinohara H, Terauchi T, et al. Multi-bed-position acquisition technique for deep inspiration breath-hold PET/CT: a preliminary result for pulmonary lesions. Ann Nucl Med 2010;24:179–88.

63. Torizuka T, Tanizaki Y, Kanno T, et al. Single 20-second acquisition of deep-inspiration breath-hold PET/CT: clinical feasibility for lung cancer. J Nucl Med 2009;50:1579–84.

64. Nagamachi S, Wakamatsu H, Kiyohara S, et al. Usefulness of a deep-inspiration breath-hold 18F-FDG PET/CT technique in diagnosing liver, bile duct, and pancreas tumors. Nucl Med Commun 2009;30:326–32.

65. Kawano T, Ohtake E, Inoue T. Deep-inspiration breath-hold PET/CT of lung cancer: maximum standardized uptake value analysis of 108 patients. J Nucl Med 2008;49:1223–31.

66. Pan T, Mawlawi O, Nehmeh SA, et al. Attenuation correction of PET images with respiration-averaged CT images in PET/CT. J Nucl Med 2005;46:1481–7.

67. Chi PC, Mawlawi O, Luo D, et al. Effects of respiration-averaged computed tomography on positron emission tomography/computed tomography quantification and its potential impact on gross tumor volume delineation. Int J Radiat Oncol Biol Phys 2008;71:890–9.

68. Meirelles GS, Erdi YE, Nehmeh SA, et al. Deep-inspiration breath-hold PET/CT: clinical findings with a new technique for detection and characterization of thoracic lesions. J Nucl Med 2007;48: 712–9.

69. Vogel WV, van Dalen JA, Wiering B, et al. Evaluation of image registration in PET/CT of the liver and recommendations for optimized imaging. J Nucl Med 2007;48:910–9.

70. Osman MM, Cohade C, Nakamoto Y, et al. Respiratory motion artifacts on PET emission images obtained using CT attenuation correction on PET-CT. Eur J Nucl Med Mol Imaging 2003;30:603–6.

71. Goerres GW, Kamel E, Seifert B, et al. Accuracy of image coregistration of pulmonary lesions in patients with non-small cell lung cancer using an integrated PET/CT system. J Nucl Med 2002;43: 1469–75.

72. Goerres GW, Kamel E, Heidelberg TN, et al. PET-CT image co-registration in the thorax: influence of respiration. Eur J Nucl Med Mol Imaging 2002; 29:351–60.

73. Beyer T, Rosenbaum S, Veit P, et al. Respiration artifacts in whole-body (18)F-FDG PET/CT studies with combined PET/CT tomographs employing spiral CT technology with 1 to 16 detector rows. Eur J Nucl Med Mol Imaging 2005;32: 1429–39.

74. Beddar AS, Briere TM, Balter P, et al. 4D-CT imaging with synchronized intravenous contrast injection to improve delineation of liver tumors for treatment planning. Radiother Oncol 2008;87(3): 445–8.

75. Gould KL, Pan T, Loghin C, et al. Frequent diagnostic errors in cardiac PET/CT due to misregistration of CT attenuation and emission PET images: a definitive analysis of causes, consequences, and corrections. J Nucl Med 2007;48:1112–21.

76. Young H, Baum R, Cremerius U, et al. Measurement of clinical and subclinical tumor response using [18F]-fluorodeoxyglucose and positron emission tomography: review and 1999 EORTC recommendations. European Organization for Research and Treatment of Cancer (EORTC) PET Study Group. Eur J Cancer 1999;35:1773–82.

77. Keall P. 4-Dimensional computed tomography imaging and treatment planning. Semin Radiat Oncol 2004;14:81–90.

78. Wahl LM, Asselin MC, Nahmias C. Regions of interest in the venous sinuses as input functions for quantitative PET. J Nucl Med 1999;40:1666–75.

79. Geworski L, Knoop BO, de Cabrejas ML, et al. Recovery correction for quantitation in emission tomography: a feasibility study. Eur J Nucl Med 2000;27:161–9.

80. Degirmenci B, Wilson D, Laymon CM, et al. Standardized uptake value-based evaluations of solitary pulmonary nodules using F-18 fluorodeoxyglucose-PET/computed tomography. Nucl Med Commun 2008;29:614–22.

81. Alessio AM, Kinahan PE, Lewellen TK. Modeling and incorporation of system response functions in 3-D whole body PET. IEEE Trans Med Imaging 2006;25:828–37.

82. Karp JS, Surti S, Daube-Witherspoon ME, et al. Benefit of time-of-flight in PET: experimental and clinical results. J Nucl Med 2008;49:462–70.

83. Soret M, Bacharach SL, Buvat I. Partial-volume effect in PET tumor imaging. J Nucl Med 2007;48: 932–45.

84. Panin VY, Kehren F, Michel C, et al. Fully 3-D PET reconstruction with system matrix derived from point source measurements. IEEE Trans Med Imaging 2006;25:907–21.

85. Qiao F, Pan T, Clark JW Jr, et al. A motion-incorporated reconstruction method for gated PET studies. Phys Med Biol 2006;51:3769–83.

86. Pan T, Lee TY, Rietzel E, et al. 4D-CT imaging of a volume influenced by respiratory motion on multi-slice CT. Med Phys 2004;31:333–40.

87. Manning K, Tepfer B, Goldklang G, et al. Clinical practice guidelines for the utilization of positron emission tomography/computed tomography imaging in selected oncologic applications: suggestions from a provider group. Mol Imaging Biol 2007;9:324–32 [discussion: 323].

88. El Naqa I, Low DA, Bradley JD, et al. Deblurring of breathing motion artifacts in thoracic PET images by deconvolution methods. Med Phys 2006;33:3587–600.

89. Werner MK, Parker JA, Kolodny GM, et al. Respiratory gating enhances imaging of pulmonary nodules and measurement of tracer uptake in FDG PET/CT. AJR Am J Roentgenol 2009;193:1640–5.

90. Rahmim A, Tang J, Zaidi H. Four-dimensional (4D) image reconstruction strategies in dynamic PET: beyond conventional independent frame reconstruction. Med Phys 2009;36:3654–70.

91. Schoenahl F, Zaidi H. Towards optimal model-based partial volume effect correction in oncological PET imaging. Proceedings of IEEE Nuclear Science Symposium & Medical Imaging Conference. Rome, Italy, October 19–22, 2004. p. 3177–81.

92. Suckling J, Ott RJ, Deehan BJ. Quantitative analysis of a reconstruction method for fully three-dimensional PET. Phys Med Biol 1992;37:751–66.

93. Townsend DW. Positron emission tomography/computed tomography. Semin Nucl Med 2008;38:152–66.

94. Rousset O, Rahmim A, Alavi A, et al. Partial volume correction strategies in PET. PET Clin 2007;2:235–49.

95. Hoffman EJ, Huang SC, Phelps ME. Quantitation in positron emission computed tomography: 1. Effect of object size. J Comput Assist Tomogr 1979;3:299–308.

96. Kessler RM, Ellis JR Jr, Eden M. Analysis of emission tomographic scan data: limitations imposed by resolution and background. J Comput Assist Tomogr 1984;8:514–22.

97. Avril N, Bense S, Ziegler SI, et al. Breast imaging with fluorine-18-FDG PET: quantitative image analysis. J Nucl Med 1997;38:1186–91.

98. Menda Y, Bushnell DL, Madsen MT, et al. Evaluation of various corrections to the standardized uptake value for diagnosis of pulmonary malignancy. Nucl Med Commun 2001;22:1077–81.

99. Hickeson M, Yun M, Matthies A, et al. Use of a corrected standardized uptake value based on the lesion size on CT permits accurate characterization of lung nodules on FDG-PET. Eur J Nucl Med Mol Imaging 2002;29:1639–47.

100. Reader AJ, Zaidi H. Advances in PET image reconstruction. PET Clinics 2007;2:173–90.

101. Da Silva AJ, Tang HR, Wong KH, et al. Absolute quantification of regional myocardial uptake of 99mTc-sestamibi with SPECT: experimental validation in a porcine model. J Nucl Med 2001;42:772–9.

102. Baete K, Nuyts J, Van Paesschen W, et al. Anatomical-based FDG-PET reconstruction for the detection of hypo-metabolic regions in epilepsy. IEEE Trans Med Imaging 2004;23:510–9.

103. Huesman RH. A new fast algorithm for the evaluation of regions of interest and statistical uncertainty in computed tomography. Phys Med Biol 1984;29:543–52.

104. Carson RE. A maximum likelihood method for region-of-interest evaluation in emission tomography. J Comput Assist Tomogr 1986;10:654–63.

105. Formiconi AR. Least squares algorithm for region of interest evaluation in emission tomography. IEEE Trans Med Imaging 1993;12:90–100.

106. Vanzi E, De Cristofaro M, Ramat S, et al. A direct ROI quantification method for inherent PVE correction: accuracy assessment in striatal SPECT measurements. Eur J Nucl Med Mol Imaging 2007;34:1480–9.

107. Baete K, Nuyts J, Van Laere K, et al. Evaluation of anatomy based reconstruction for partial volume correction in brain FDG-PET. Neuroimage 2004;23:305–17.

108. Zaidi H, Ojha N, Morich M, et al. PET performance of the Ingenuity TF PET-MR: a whole body PET-MRI system. Phys Med Biol 2011;56:3091–106.

109. Teo BK, Seo Y, Bacharach SL, et al. Partial-volume correction in PET: validation of an iterative postreconstruction method with phantom and patient data. J Nucl Med 2007;48:802–10.

110. Qiao F, Pan T, Clark JW Jr, et al. Joint model of motion and anatomy for PET image reconstruction. Med Phys 2007;34:4626–39.

111. Boussion N, Cheze Le Rest C, Hatt M, et al. Incorporation of wavelet-based denoising in iterative deconvolution for partial volume correction in whole-body PET imaging. Eur J Nucl Med Mol Imaging 2009;36:1064–75.

112. Chen CH, Muzic RF Jr, Nelson AD, et al. Simultaneous recovery of size and radioactivity concentration of small spheroids with PET data. J Nucl Med 1999;40:118–30.

113. Evans PM. Anatomical imaging for radiotherapy. Phys Med Biol 2008;53:R151–91.

114. Perez CA. Principles and practice of radiation oncology. 4th edition. Lippincott Williams & Wilkins, Philadelphia; 2004.

115. Basu S. Selecting the optimal image segmentation strategy in the era of multitracer multimodality imaging: a critical step for image-guided radiation therapy. Eur J Nucl Med Mol Imaging 2009;36: 180–1.

116. Boudraa A, Zaidi H. Image segmentation techniques in nuclear medicine imaging. In: Zaidi H, editor. Quantitative analysis of nuclear medicine images. New York: Springer; 2006. p. 308–57.

117. Boudraa A, Cexus JC, Zaidi H. Functional segmentation of dynamic nuclear medicine images by cross-PsiB energy operator. Comput Meth Prog Biomed 2006;84:148–54.

118. Kiffer JD, Berlangieri SU, Scott AM, et al. The contribution of 18F-fluoro-2-deoxy-glucose positron emission tomographic imaging to radiotherapy planning in lung cancer. Lung Cancer 1998;19:167–77.

119. Wang H, Vees H, Miralbell R, et al. 18F-choline PET-based target volume delineation techniques for partial prostate reirradiation in local recurrent prostate cancer. Radiother Oncol 2009;93:220–5.

120. Zaidi H. Medical image segmentation: Quo Vadis. Comput Meth Prog Biomed 2006;84:63–7.

121. Jannin P, Krupinski E, Warfield S. Guest editorial validation in medical image processing. IEEE Trans Med Imaging 2006;25:1405–9.

122. Slomka P, Baum R. Multimodality image registration with software: state-of-the-art. Eur J Nucl Med Mol Imaging 2009;36:44–55.

123. Belhassen S, Llina Fuentes CS, Dekker A, et al. Comparative methods for 18F-FDG PET-based delineation of target volumes in non-small-cell lung cancer [abstract]. J Nucl Med 2009;50:27P.

124. Daisne JF, Sibomana M, Bol A, et al. Tri-dimensional automatic segmentation of PET volumes based on measured source-to-background ratios: influence of reconstruction algorithms. Radiother Oncol 2003;69:247–50.

125. Graves EE, Quon A, Loo BW Jr. RT_Image: an open-source tool for investigating PET in radiation oncology. Technol Cancer Res Treat 2007;6:111–21.

126. Black QC, Grills IS, Kestin LL, et al. Defining a radiotherapy target with positron emission tomography. Int J Radiat Oncol Biol Phys 2004; 60:1272–82.

127. Nestle U, Kremp S, Schaefer-Schuler A, et al. Comparison of different methods for delineation of 18F-FDG PET-positive tissue for target volume definition in radiotherapy of patients with non-Small cell lung cancer. J Nucl Med 2005;46: 1342–8.

128. Boudraa AE, Champier J, Cinotti L, et al. Delineation and quantitation of brain lesions by fuzzy clustering in positron emission tomography. Comput Med Imaging Graph 1996;20:31–41.

129. Belhassen S, Zaidi H. A novel fuzzy C-means algorithm for unsupervised heterogeneous tumor quantification in PET. Med Phys 2010;37:1309–24.

Index

PET Clin 6 (2011) 227–229
doi:10.1016/S1556-8598(11)00056-3

Moving?

Make sure your subscription moves with you!

To notify us of your new address, find your **Clinics Account Number** (located on your mailing label above your name), and contact customer service at:

Email: journalscustomerservice-usa@elsevier.com

800-654-2452 (subscribers in the U.S. & Canada)
314-447-8871 (subscribers outside of the U.S. & Canada)

Fax number: 314-447-8029

Elsevier Health Sciences Division
Subscription Customer Service
3251 Riverport Lane
Maryland Heights, MO 63043

*To ensure uninterrupted delivery of your subscription, please notify us at least 4 weeks in advance of move.

ELSEVIER

Printed and bound by CPI Group (UK) Ltd, Croydon, CR0 4YY

03/10/2024

01040348-0013